THE NEW
MEDITERRANEAN
DIET COOKBOOK

THE OPTIMAL KETO-FRIENDLY DIET THAT BURNS FAT, PROMOTES LONGEVITY, AND PREVENTS CHRONIC DISEASE

Martina Slajerova ✦ Dr. Nicholas Norwitz

Thomas DeLauer ✦ Rohan Kashid

FAIR WINDS

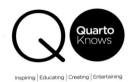

Inspiring | Educating | Creating | Entertaining

Brimming with creative inspiration, how-to projects, and useful information to enrich your everyday life, Quarto Knows is a favorite destination for those pursuing their interests and passions. Visit our site and dig deeper with our books into your area of interest: Quarto Creates, Quarto Cooks, Quarto Homes, Quarto Lives, Quarto Drives, Quarto Explores, Quarto Gifts, or Quarto Kids.

First Published in 2021 by Fair Winds Press, an imprint of The Quarto Group, 100 Cummings Center, Suite 265-D, Beverly, MA 01915, USA.
T (978) 282-9590 F (978) 283-2742 QuartoKnows.com

Fair Winds Press titles are also available at discount for retail, wholesale, promotional, and bulk purchase. For details, contact the Special Sales Manager by email at specialsales@quarto.com or by mail at The Quarto Group, Attn: Special Sales Manager, 100 Cummings Center, Suite 265-D, Beverly, MA 01915, USA.

24 23 22 21   4

ISBN: 978-1-58923-991-3

Digital edition published in 2021
eISBN: 978-1-58923-992-0

Library of Congress Cataloging-in-Publication Data available.

Design: Megan Jones Design
Cover Image: Martina Slajerova
Page Layout: Megan Jones Design
Photography: Martina Slajerova and Jo Harding
Illustration: Eleanor Stanton

Printed in China

The information in this book is for educational purposes only. It is not intended to replace the advice of a physician or medical practitioner. Please see your healthcare provider before beginning any new health program.

Health is a lifelong journey that requires support.
Each author would like to dedicate this book to one special
person who has helped them on their health journeys:

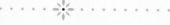

MARTINA SLAJEROVA:

I would like to dedicate this book to my soul
mate and my best friend, Nikos, who has
always inspired, supported, and encouraged
me throughout my health journey.

DR. NICHOLAS NORWITZ:

I dedicate this book to Dr. Vyvane Loh,
who not only saved my life by showing
me the power of metabolic medicine
and food, but who also has since
become my adopted second mother.

THOMAS DELAUER:

I would like to dedicate this book to
my father, who passed away of cancer.
It is truly because of him that I decided
to try my hardest to make my voice
heard on the topic of health.

ROHAN KASHID:

My dedication goes to my loving
grandfather, who died of Alzheimer's disease.
In his memory, I hope that this book can
contribute a small part to the prevention
of this devastating condition.

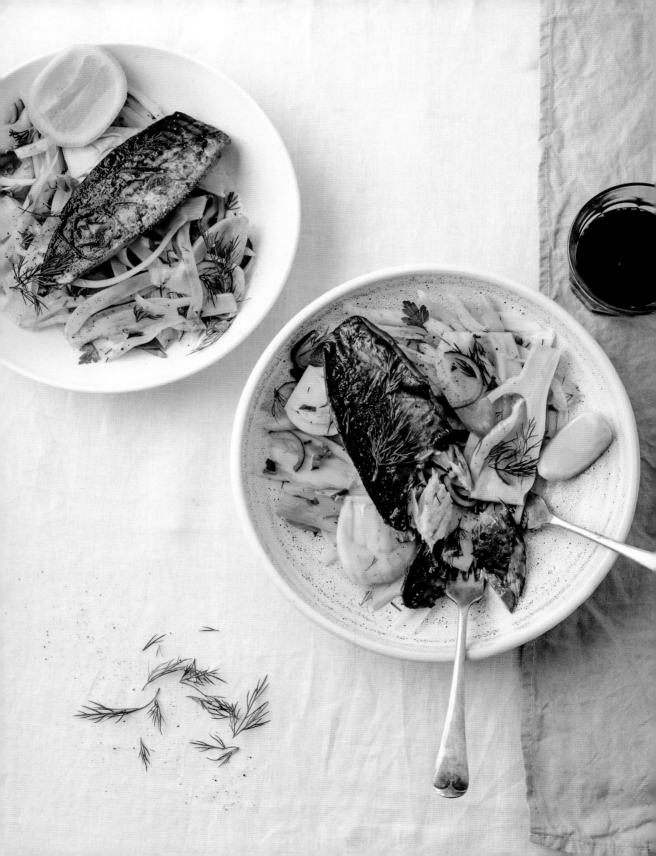

CONTENTS

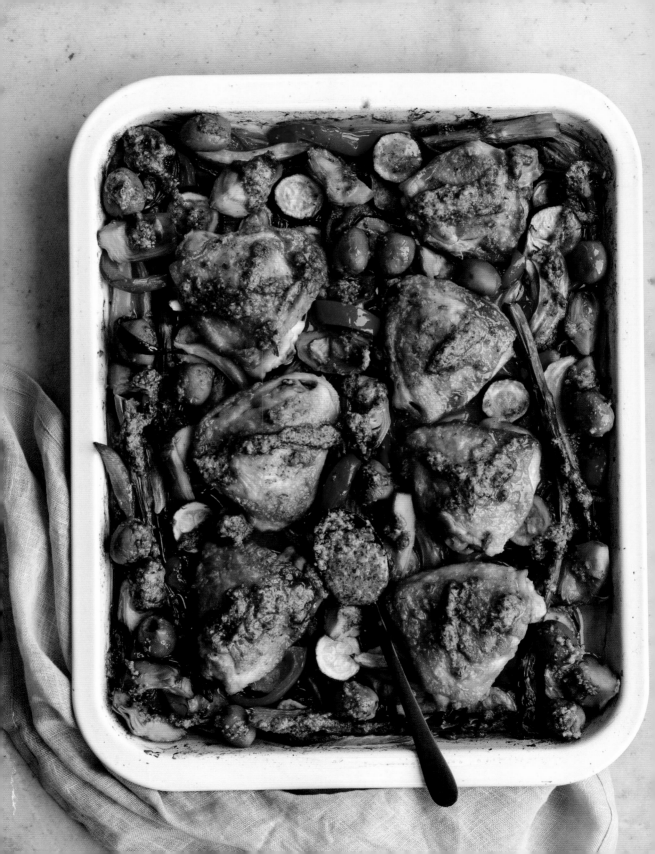

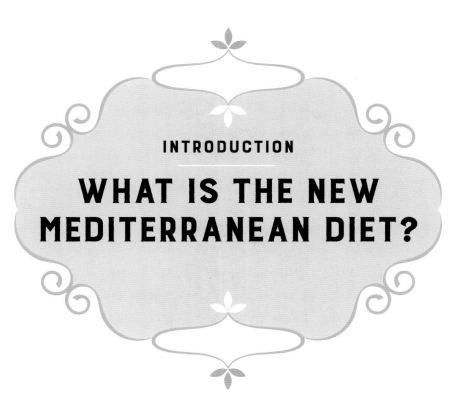

INTRODUCTION

WHAT IS THE NEW MEDITERRANEAN DIET?

Simply put, the New Mediterranean Diet is a forward-looking culinary method that blends cutting-edge science with delicious food to optimize health, wellness, and longevity. This book is based on two principles: First, that good food is the foundation of good health; and second, that science is a tool we can use in the kitchen to maximize nutrition in our meals.

We, the authors of *The New Mediterranean Diet Cookbook*, are a team of chefs, scientists, and health care providers who collectively possess decades of experience—in the kitchen and in laboratories, hospitals, and other settings that focus on caring for people with chronic diseases. We hope that this book will guide you to build healthy meals at home and that it will transform your kitchen into the most important room in your house: a meeting point for science, nutrition, and great taste.

Welcome to being a chef and a scientist! And, most importantly, *bon appétit!*

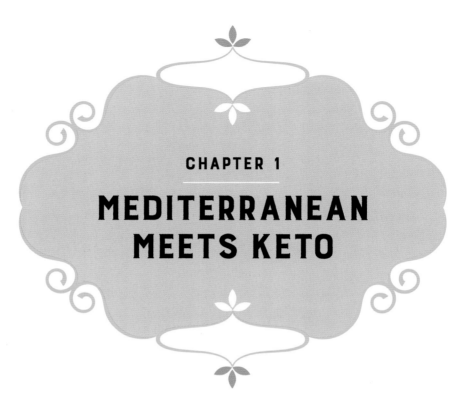

CHAPTER 1

MEDITERRANEAN MEETS KETO

Science is all about developing models—or ways of understanding the world—that are tested, tweaked, and retested continuously as new evidence emerges. As a science-based cookbook, this book follows the same approach. In the spirit of science, let's start at the very beginning. What is the starting model upon which *The New Mediterranean Diet Cookbook* is founded?

Well, there are actually two foundations to our approach: Mediterranean diets and ketogenic diets, both of which have advantages. Mediterranean diets are associated with leanness, longevity, and lower rates of the age-related chronic diseases that plague modern society, including obesity, diabetes, heart disease, and Alzheimer's. And an increasing body of evidence suggests that low-carb, high-fat ketogenic diets can also promote healthy body weight and fight these same chronic diseases.

So why choose just one? You certainly don't have to! Mediterranean diets and ketogenic diets are often cast as mutually exclusive, but they are actually perfectly complementary styles of eating. While Mediterranean diets are all about food sources, ketogenic diets are all about balancing macronutrients (that is, keeping a close eye on how much fat, carbs, and protein you consume).

Think of it this way: Mediterranean diets are about *what* you eat, while ketogenic diets are about *how much* you eat. That means they can work in tandem (if you're mathematically inclined, you could call them perpendicular), and that you can get the best of both worlds by eating a Mediterranean-ketogenic diet.

The concept of Mediterranean-keto is just the starting point for this book. Guided by the latest science, it can be further tweaked, optimized, and developed into something even better—what we call "the New Mediterranean Diet."

HEALTH SCIENCE YOU SHOULD KNOW

Science is never static: its process depends upon change, revision, and redevelopment. The same is true for the New Mediterranean Diet. That's why it's so important that you don't just take us at our word in this book but attempt to *learn* (and hopefully get excited!) about nutrition science and your own personal health journey.

To help you with that, recipes in this book come with fun facts! But before we get to the recipes, in the following four sections we'll give you a crash course on some of the science that underpins the recipes:

- A nibble of evidence supporting the health claims of Mediterranean and ketogenic diets.

- An explanation of some key vocabulary terms that appear throughout this book; understanding them will benefit your health and well-being.

- A descriptive list of the New Mediterranean staple foods you'll rely on as you cook your way through this book, including seven high-fat superfoods!

- A guide to understanding recipe nutrition.

While you could skip any one of these sections—just as you *could* skip the soup, salad, or appetizer when you're having a meal—we recommend you read on in order to fully appreciate your New Mediterranean experience.

WHAT'S THE EVIDENCE?

In this book's subtitle, we state that the New Mediterranean Diet "burns fats, promotes longevity, and prevents chronic disease." Here's some evidence for those claims:

- **Burns fat.** In a landmark study, forty overweight people were split into two groups. Although both groups consumed the same number of calories, one group followed a ketogenic diet, while the other ate a low-fat diet. After three months, the keto diet group had, on average, lost more than twice as much weight (24 pounds) as the low-fat group (11 pounds). And that's not all! Although the keto group *ate more than twice as much fat* as the low-fat folks, the *fat in their blood decreased by 150 percent more* than the low-fat eaters! Why? Because their bodies were burning fat as energy!

- **Promotes longevity.** The Mediterranean region is a Blue Zone, an area of the world in which people tend to live much longer than average. It's generally assumed that this longevity is, in part, due to the extra-virgin olive oil, fish, and vegetable-rich diets enjoyed by Mediterranean people. While the assumption that a Mediterranean diet will enhance longevity is mostly based on human epidemiology (association) studies, studies conducted on mice have produced complementary results to support the notion that ketogenic diets enhance longevity and health. In a 2017 study published in the prestigious journal *Cell Metabolism*, researchers discovered that putting mice on a ketogenic diet increased their life spans by 13 percent! Plus, unlike mice fed a standard, carb-rich diet, the "ketogenic mice" maintained both their physical fitness and cognitive function into old age. Nobody is yet sure what the results of combining Mediterranean and keto diets in humans will be, but judging from this and other research, eating this way will probably increase your chances of being around to find out!

- **Fights chronic disease.** If current trends continue as projected, a staggering one-third of Americans will be type II diabetic by 2050. Until recently, diabetes was considered a progressive and irreversible condition. However, new science is challenging the status quo. A 2019 study compared the effects of a two-year ketogenic diet to the standard of care, which involved medications, check-ins with primary care physicians or endocrinologists, and nutritional recommendations based on the American Diabetes Association from registered dieticians. Astonishingly, the ketogenic diet completely reversed type II diabetes in

54 percent of the 262 ketogenic patients who took part in the study. What's more, 60 percent of the ketogenic diet patients were able to discontinue their use of insulin. By comparison, the overall condition of patients in the standard of care group worsened, and almost all had to increase their insulin doses.

KEY VOCABULARY TERMS

Science is filled with intimidating jargon, but most of it can be made much easier to digest (pun intended!) and much more fun to read. Take a look at this sentence, for example: "Pink-red salmon contain antioxidants and fats that are particularly good for brain health" rather than—brace yourself—"Salmon, particularly *Oncorhynchus nerka*, contain astaxanthin, an amphipathic antioxidant capable of blood-brain barrier penetration and electron dislocation resonance, which functions to diminish the oxidation of *O. nerka*'s 22:6 (n-3) docosahexaenoic acid fraction, yielding a high-integrity form of the brain's main structural lipid substrate." Are you asleep yet?

Don't worry, you won't come across complicated lingo like that in this book! That said, there are a few key terms you'll want to know. Hopefully, these analogies help! Specifically, you should understand the concepts of (1) Oxidative Stress, (2) Inflammation, (3) Insulin, (4) Fatty Acids, and (5) LDL Cholesterol:

① **Oxidative Stress:** *The bull in the china shop.* Cells turn nutrients into energy that our bodies can use. As a result of this process, cells produce toxic by-products called "reactive oxygen species." Think of them as bulls in the proverbial china shop, except here the china shop is the tiny cell. Reactive oxygen species bounce around and damage everything in their way, even your DNA!

Oxidative Stress

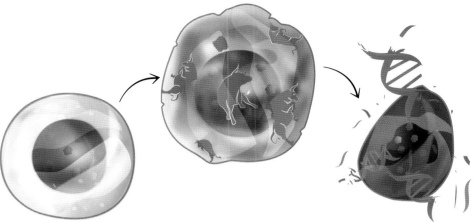

This harmful bouncing-around process is called "oxidative stress."

- **Antioxidants:** Molecules—some found in your body and some eaten in food—that neutralize reactive oxygen species and defend against oxidative stress.

- **Polyphenol:** A group of antioxidants found in food such as colorful veggies, dark chocolate, and extra-virgin olive oil.

② **Inflammation:** *The overeager soldiers.* Your immune system is like an army, a group of soldiers defending your body from marauding infections. Although inflammation is part of the normal healing process—say, when you have a wound or a broken bone—when the inflammation goes on for too long, it can damage body tissues, such as the brain, and lead to disease. Our modern diets and lifestyles often unnecessarily activate our immune systems, damaging cells—we call this "chronic inflammation." Chronic inflammation is toxic, and, sadly, so common in modern Western society that most doctors and scientists just call it "inflammation."

- **Anti-inflammatory:** A property of molecules that helps prevent or reduce inflammation. Most antioxidants are also anti-inflammatory.

Inflammation

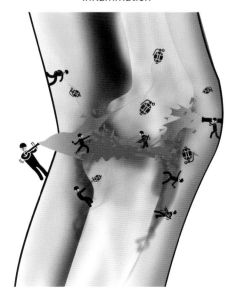

③ **Insulin:** *The inky octopus.* Insulin is a hormone with more vital functions than an octopus has arms. Insulin helps muscles grow, increases cardiac efficiency, and is important for brain health. However, like an octopus that squirts you with ink, insulin has a naughty side, too. When agitated by the consumption of carbs, insulin sticks to fat cells, causing them to grow. Plus, when it does this, the octopus—that is, insulin—soon shirks its important duties, like the abovementioned ones. This is insulin resistance, a state in which the body experiences more of the fat-producing effects of insulin and fewer of its benefits. But there's good news: If you don't poke the insulin octopus with too many carbs, you won't get squirted with ink. A great reason to keep your fingers out of the donut tank!

Insulin Resistance

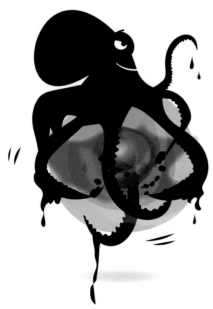

When agitated by carbs, the insulin octopus suctions onto fat cells and causes them to grow. If insulin had ink, it would be miracle grow for fat cells.

Fatty Acids

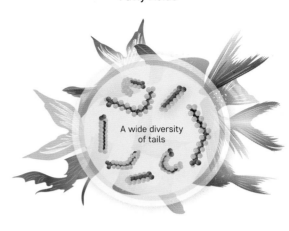

A wide diversity of tails

④ **Fatty Acids:** *Fish with straight and bendy tails.* The different types of fat we eat contain fatty acids, microscopic tail-like chemical structures. Differences among fatty-acid tails, including length and bends, determine the nutritional properties of different fats.

- **Saturated & Unsaturated:** Saturated fats have straight tails with no bends. Unsaturated fats have bendy tails. Saturated fats are more stable, which can actually be a good thing because it means they are more resistant to damage by oxidative stress. On the other hand, many unsaturated fats are also beneficial, such as "MUFA" and omega-3s.

- **Monounsaturated (MUFA) & Polyunsaturated (PUFA) Fats:** These are types of unsaturated fats. MUFAs have one tail bend. They are quite stable like saturated fats, but also have beneficial signaling properties that can help improve metabolic health. Mediterranean diets are rich in sources of MUFAs—think extra-virgin olive oil, avocados, and macadamia nuts.

- **Omega-3 & Omega-6 Fats:** There are different types of PUFAs, including omega-3 and omega-6 fats. Omega-3 fats are found mostly in seafood and are anti-inflammatory. Too many omega-6 fats, particularly those from processed foods, can promote inflammation.

- **Omega-6/3 Ratio:** Most of us consume too many omega-6-rich foods and too few omega-3 foods. This leads to a high omega-6/3 ratio and ultimately promotes oxidative stress and chronic inflammation.

⑤ **Lipoproteins, Cholesterol, Triglycerides:**
The boats in your bloodstream. Low-density-lipoprotein (LDL) is like a boat that transports two types of cargo through the bloodstream. LDL transports cholesterol (an essential building block for cell membranes and hormones) and triglycerides (fat fuel) from the liver to organs around the body that need building blocks and fuel.

LDL levels can increase for two reasons. First, if you're eating a ketogenic or low-carb diet and burning fat as fuel, your liver may send out more LDL "boats" to supply fat fuel to your muscles. The empty LDL boats return to the liver to dock, restock, and go back to work. The second reason is more sinister: When you overeat carbs, it's as if you're filling your bloodstream with sugar glaciers. The LDL boats bump into these sugar glaciers and get damaged in a process called "glycation." Glycation, in turn, makes those LDL boats further vulnerable to oxidative stress. Once they've been damaged by the sugar glaciers, the LDL boats can't return to the liver and end up accumulating in your bloodstream. Eventually, they sink down to your artery walls and develop into atherosclerotic plaques, a titanic health catastrophe.

Therefore, the perception that LDL is "bad" is not entirely true. Having more LDL in your bloodstream may be necessary when you're burning lots of fat fuel. However, LDL is bad when it gets damaged by carbs and oxidation, because then it may contribute to heart disease.

Finally, there's "high-density lipoprotein" (HDL). Often called "good" cholesterol, HDL is like a rescue submarine that salvages cargo from sinking LDL, cleaning up your bloodstream, and protecting against heart disease.

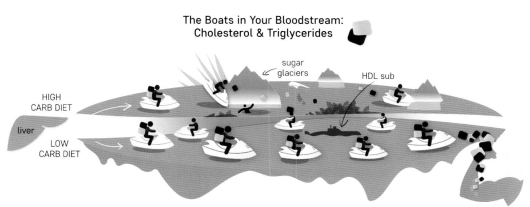

The Boats in Your Bloodstream:
Cholesterol & Triglycerides

sugar glaciers

HDL sub

HIGH CARB DIET

liver

LOW CARB DIET

On a low-carb diet, your liver may send out more LDL boats to supply your muscles with energy because you're burning fat for fuel.

NEW MEDITERRANEAN STAPLE FOODS

SEVEN HIGH-FAT SUPERFOODS

Now that you've learned why eating at the inter-section of Mediterranean and ketogenic diets is great for your health and you've gotten a few key scientific vocabulary terms under your belt, it's time to meet our superfoods!

① Salmon & Other Fatty Fish

DEEP DIVE

Salmon is rich in protein and micronutrients, and it's also a particularly rich source of the omega-3 fat, docosahexaenoic acid (DHA). DHA is arguably the most beneficial form of the three omega-3 fatty acids (ALA, EPA, and DHA) because of the role it plays in brain health. DHA makes up a large fraction of the brain, and routine DHA consumption promotes brain development in fetuses and

protects against cognitive decline. DHA truly benefits the brain from womb to tomb!

Salmon is also rich in astaxanthin, one of the world's best disease-fighting antioxidants. It is powerful, with six hundred times the antioxidant capacity of blueberries and six thousand times (yes, you read that right!) the antioxidant capacity of vitamin C. It can also neutralize up to twenty different toxic "free radicals" simultaneously (remember the bull in the cellular china shop on page 10)?

Most important, astaxanthin is both water- and fat-soluble, meaning it can reach every part of the body, from your blood to the inside of cells to your brain! This last property is particularly beneficial because the brain super-fat, DHA, is vulnerable to being destroyed by oxidation.

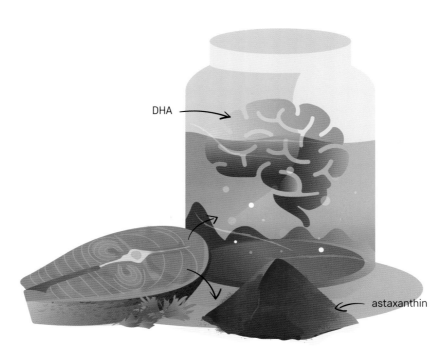

DHA

astaxanthin

Therefore, salmon not only provides a dose of the most important brain fat, but also supplies an ideal way to defend it from harm! Impressive, right?

Because astaxanthin from salmon can reach every part of the body, its health benefits are far-reaching. Evidence suggests that astaxanthin can help prevent cancers, inflammatory diseases, metabolic syndrome, type II diabetes, heart disease, gastrointestinal diseases, liver diseases, neurodegenerative diseases, eye diseases, skin diseases, and maybe even wrinkles too.

 PRACTICAL TIP

Astaxanthin gives salmon its beautiful red-pink color! Salmon acquire astaxanthin from eating red-pink krill and swimming upstream, against currents. This is a major reason for buying wild, not farmed, salmon. Look for wild Alaskan sockeye, if you can find it—it's the best variety. Remember: The redder, the better!

 KEY POINTS

① Salmon and other fatty fish are rich in the fat DHA, which is important for brain health.

② Salmon contain the red-pink pigment astaxanthin, a powerful antioxidant that fights disease.

③ Wild Alaskan sockeye contain the most astaxanthin.

② Extra-Virgin Olive Oil (EVOO)

DEEP DIVE

Justifiably, the abbreviation for extra-virgin olive oil sounds like a cry of triumph: *EVOO!* The history of EVOO is very interesting. Not only did Athena, the Greek goddess of wisdom, supposedly bestow olives on the Greeks, but EVOO was also the monetary currency of the ancient Greeks' predecessors, the Minoans. Since the Greeks invented democracy, can we credit EVOO with developing modern civilization?

But the value of EVOO surpasses legend and economics. EVOO is the archetypal high-fat superfood, rich in oleic acid, a type of heart-healthy MUFA. The right dose of oleic acid can decrease oxidative stress and inflammation, and generally protect against chronic diseases. But oleic acid is more than a superb fatty fuel; it's also the precursor of a signaling molecule called oleoylethanolamine (OEA). By activating DNA-controlling proteins (PPAR transcription factors), OEA from EVOO increases fat metabolism. OEA also binds to receptors on the vagus nerve that connects the gut to the brain. In response, the brain releases oxytocin, the "cuddle and fullness" hormone. Therefore, the oleic acid in EVOO can increase fat burning and decrease the hunger drive.

But what really makes EVOO stand out is that it's packed with at least thirty-six antioxidant polyphenols, such as hydroxytyrosol and oleocanthal. Hydroxytyrosol is renowned as one of the most powerful natural antioxidants (right up there with astaxanthin from salmon), boasting ten times the antioxidant power of green tea! A large body of evidence suggests that hydroxytyrosol from EVOO may protect against atherosclerosis and heart disease, osteoporosis, macular degeneration, metabolic syndrome, cancers, and neurodegenerative diseases.

Oleocanthal is another nutrient superstar. It may help the brain clean up amyloid oligomers and prevents tau fibrillization, which are two toxic molecules that are thought to contribute to cognitive decline. Amyloid and tau are the hallmarks of Alzheimer's disease. So, it's your call, "Where did I put my keys?" or "*EVOO! . . .* They're in your pocket."

EVOOs should be cold-pressed (and from the first press) of the olive to retain nutritional integrity. When buying, you'll need to choose wisely: 80 percent of EVOOs don't meet these standards, and some are even diluted with other oils. To get the benefits of oleic acid, OEA, hydroxytyrosol, oleocanthal, and the other thirty-four polyphenols found in EVOO, you need to buy from the correct 20 percent of the market.

PRACTICAL TIP

Here are four steps to choosing real EVOO:

① Examine the bottle. If it is not made from dark glass or metal, the oil isn't being protected from oxidation.

② Check the label for a "pressed," "harvested," or "crushed" date. Good dealers want to demonstrate that their oil was produced within the last eighteen months.

③ Note the price. EVOO is expensive to make. If a bottle is less than $10 for 500 mL, it's probably fake.

④ Do a taste test. Oleocanthal binds to TRPA1 receptors in the back of the throat to cause a peppery sting. If you take a sip of EVOO and get a sting, it suggests oleocanthal and other polyphenols are present. That's why the best EVOOs are called "two-cough" oils—their sting makes you cough twice.

KEY POINTS

① The body makes OEA—a fat-burning, fullness-causing molecule—from the oleic acid in EVOO.

② EVOO's polyphenols prevent oxidative stress and inflammation, which cause chronic diseases.

③ Eighty percent of oils labeled as EVOO are fake. To choose the right EVOO, follow the four tips above.

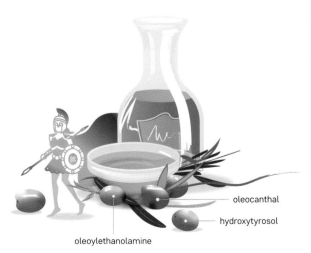

oleocanthal

hydroxytyrosol

oleoylethanolamine

③ **Avocado & Avocado Oil**

DEEP DIVE

Avocados epitomize the logic behind "food as medicine." Whole foods are complex ecosystems of nutrients that add up to be healthier than the sum of their parts. This couldn't be more true than for the humble avocado, also known as the "butter pear" or the "Da Vinci Food." (Okay, the "Da Vinci Food" is ours. We hope it catches on.)

Avocados are well known for the healthy fats they contain, specifically oleic acid, which we discussed in conjunction with EVOO. This means that avocado fat confers similar health benefits to EVOO fat, decreasing oxidative stress and inflammation, activating fat-burning genes, and stimulating the vagus nerve to make you feel full. Furthermore, avocado oil stands out among healthy MUFA sources in that it has a high smoke point, suggesting that avocado oil should be a go-to cooking oil. Avocados are also packed with prebiotic fibers, vitamins, and minerals, including vitamins B_6 and K_1, folate, magnesium, and potassium. One avocado berry (yes, avocados are actually berries) contains more potassium than two large bananas!

Just as Leonardo da Vinci's talents aren't confined to the *Mona Lisa*, there is more to the avocado than meets the eye. Apart from vitamins and minerals, avocados contain more than a hundred bioactive compounds (from inflammation-fighting anthocyanidins to vision-boosting zeaxanthin) that collectively protect the heart and brain, kill off viruses and parasites, decrease

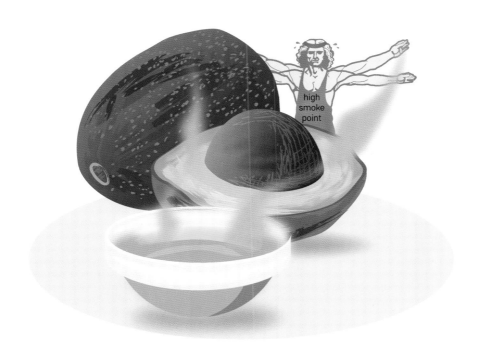

high smoke point

inflammation, promote gut health, and even kill cancer cells. Here's just one example: Two "randomized, blinded, placebo-controlled, crossover" human studies (the gold standard in nutrition science) found that eating one avocado per day lowers the two most atherogenic (cardiovascular disease-causing) forms of LDL cholesterol—small dense and oxidized LDLs—thus preventing heart disease! Remember our LDL boats (page 13)?

Best of all, avocados are nutrient multipliers for other vegetables with which they are usually paired. For example, adding avocado to salad increases the body's absorption of the carotenoid β-carotene (pro-vitamin A) by 1,500 percent and increases blood levels of HDL3, which transports the brain- and vision-boosting compound lutein to where it's needed in the brain and eyes. Their ability to enhance the absorption of nutrients comes in large part from their fattiness. Remember, fat is our friend, and avocados offer a lovely way to add healthy fats to our diets. It's a wonderful culinary coincidence that avocados are so versatile—they serve as base ingredients for many dishes in this book.

④ Macadamia Nuts & Macadamia Oil

DEEP DIVE

Macadamia are the King of Nuts, a snack fit for royalty! Maybe that's why Great Britain's Queen Elizabeth, the world's longest-reigning living monarch, eats a handful a day! Macadamia nuts are special, and different from other nuts, for three reasons. First, they contain little to no inflammatory omega-6 fats. Second, they are the only type of nut nearly free from phytic acid, a plant anti-nutrient that can bind to essential minerals, such as calcium, in the gut to block their absorption. And, finally, they're the lowest in carbs.

But macadamia's superiority over other nuts isn't all they've got going for them. Macadamia stand out for their astonishingly healthy fat profile. They are the world's richest natural source of healthy MUFAs, which, as you know, are also found in olive and avocado oils. And among these three super-MUFA-rich fats sources, only macadamia is almost entirely absent of inflammatory omega-6 fats.

Above all else, though, it is palmitoleic acid that makes macadamia truly "mac-nificent." Compelling research demonstrates that this extremely rare omega-7 fat (found in high levels only in macadamia and a bitter plant called sea buckthorn) is more than just an ideal fuel—it's also a powerful signaling molecule that attaches to receptors in cells to change metabolism! In human studies, palmitoleic acid has been shown to decrease inflammation, blood fat, and bad forms of LDL cholesterol by as much as 44 percent, thus preventing heart disease. It also improves insulin sensitivity and remarkably increases levels of the fullness hormone cholecystokinin, helping to protect against type II diabetes, metabolic syndrome, and obesity.

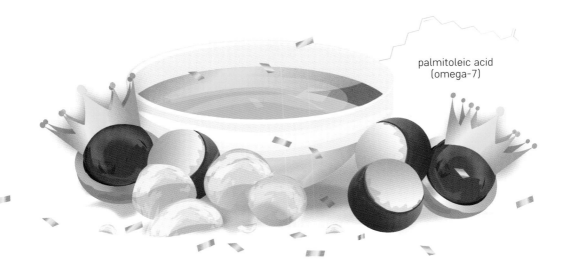

palmitoleic acid
(omega-7)

PRACTICAL TIPS

① Research suggests that eating just fifteen macadamia nuts per day is enough to reap many of their cardiovascular benefits!

② To achieve an optimal balance between your dietary sources of healthy MUFAs, use avocado oil for cooking and a mixture of extra-virgin olive oil and macadamia nut oil elsewhere.

KEY POINTS

① Macadamia are the King of Nuts because they are basically free from the anti-nutrient phytic acid, inflammatory omega-6 fats, and carbs.

② Macadamia nuts and oil are the richest natural source of MUFAs. They even beat olive oil!

③ Macadamia nuts and oil are a unique source of the rare omega-7 fat, palmitoleic acid. Palmitoleic acid is a super fuel and a powerful health-promoting "lipokine" hormone that can protect against heart disease, type II diabetes, metabolic syndrome, obesity, and many more chronic diseases.

⑤ Dark Chocolate & Cacao

DEEP DIVE

You may not be surprised to learn that the cacao beans used to make chocolate come from the *Theobroma cacao* tree, which translates as "food of the gods." But chocolate's nutritional divinity depends on how much it's been processed. Therefore, it's important to be informed about the journey of chocolate, from bean to bar.

Once cacao beans have been harvested, fermented, and dried, they can be roasted, at which point they are no longer called "cacao," but become "cocoa." Roasted cocoa can be crushed into "nibs," ground into "baker's chocolate," and melted into "liquor." The liquor is separated into fat and powder, called "cocoa butter" and "cocoa mass," respectively. The butter and mass are recombined with sugar to make chocolate bars of different "percentages." To make a long story short, all this processing eliminates nutrients. Thus, it's best to buy as far up the chain as possible or look for "high-flavanol" chocolate or cacao powder.

Cacao "flavanols" are antioxidant, anti-inflammatory molecules that contribute to many of chocolate's amazing health benefits. Just 2 ounces (57 g) of high-flavanol dark chocolate can decrease blood pressure and increase blood flow to the heart. Cacao and its flavanols also prevent the development of atherogenic plaques, increase good HDL cholesterol, and decrease LDL oxidation.

In addition to protecting the heart, chocolate also protects the brain by increasing cerebral blood flow, increasing levels of growth factors like brain-derived neurotrophic factor (BDNF), which helps brain cells renew and regenerate, and combating the amyloid oligomer toxicity that contributes to Alzheimer's disease. In one study, when a rat model of Alzheimer's disease ate 70 percent high-flavanol dark chocolate, their cognitive performance improved.

As a fermented food, like kimchi, chocolate is also prebiotic—it feeds healthy gut bacteria and decreases inflammation. And it's rich in the "love molecule" phenethylamine, which is used to treat depression. In fact (after adjusting for confounding factors such as age, BMI, and sugar intake), dark chocolate consumption (but not milk or white chocolate consumption) has been associated with a 70 percent reduced risk of depression. So be kind to your mind and eat some chocolate that's unrefined!

 PRACTICAL TIP

The amount of chocolate you should consume depends on its flavanol content. If you buy cacao or a product with a label that says "high-flavanol," 1 to 2 ounces (28 to 57 g) may be enough to get the heart, brain, and gut benefits.

 KEY POINTS

① "Cacao" is the most natural form of chocolate and confers the greatest health benefits. Alternatively, you can buy "high-flavanol" cocoa and chocolate.

② Dark chocolate is naturally low-carb and is packed with anti-inflammatory micronutrients.

③ An impressive body of evidence suggests that the unique cocktail of compounds in chocolate can reduce the risk of heart disease, protect the brain, improve gut health, treat inflammatory disorders, and enhance mood.

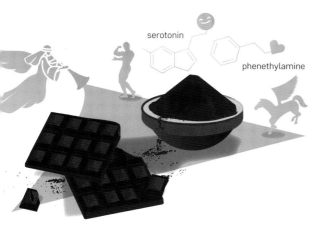

serotonin

phenethylamine

⑥ Sesame

DEEP DIVE

By now, you know that a Mediterranean diet is rich in healthy MUFA sources such as EVOO, avocado, and macadamia nuts. You also know that omega-6 PUFA sources tend to be inflammatory and should be eaten in moderation. Well, sesame is equal parts MUFA and omega-6—but unlike other major sources of omega-6, it is powerfully anti-inflammatory.

The reason sesame seeds, sesame oil, and sesame butter (tahini) break the "omega-6 fat sources are inflammatory" rule is that they are also rich in three special antioxidant, anti-inflammatory molecules, which we call the Terrific Trio:

sesamin, sesamolin, and sesamol. Research shows that as little as 1.5 ounces (40 g) of sesame per day can decrease oxidative stress and inflammation and the symptoms of certain inflammatory diseases, such as osteoarthritis. By boosting the brain's antioxidant power, sesame can even protect against cognitive decline in animal models.

Finally, DNA studies show that the Terrific Trio increases the production of fat-burning ("β-oxidation") and alcohol-metabolizing ("alcohol dehydrogenase") proteins by as much as 410 percent, meaning sesame's Terrific Trio may literally help your body burn fat and process alcohol!

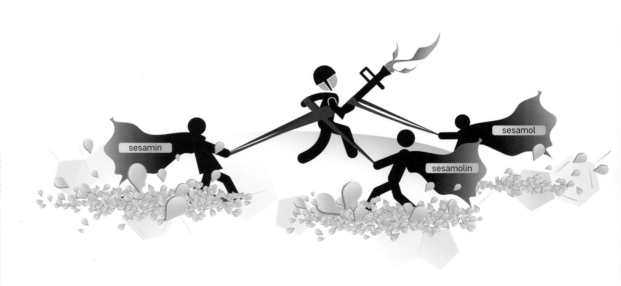

⑦ Coconut

DEEP DIVE

Coconut is controversial. In contrast to the other six high-fat superfoods in this section, it stands out for being low in MUFA and rich in saturated fat. As Mediterranean diets are known for being rich in MUFA and relatively low in saturated fat—and because saturated fats are still often (unfairly) maligned as unhealthy—we think it's important to justify our inclusion of coconut here.

Not all saturated fats are created equal. Fat "saturation" only refers to the presence or absence of bends in a fat's tail (see the discussion of fatty acids on page 12). Fats also vary in tail length. Compared to saturated animal fats, coconut fats have shorter tails and are processed differently by your body. While longer-tailed saturated fats are sent directly from your gut to your main blood circulation, about 70 percent of coconut's fats get sent directly to the liver, where they can be used immediately as clean cellular fuel.

The source of the Coconut Controversy comes down to two nuanced points that tend to get lost in the scientific literature. First, there is an important difference between "refined" and "virgin" coconut oil. When oil is refined, it loses about 85 percent of its disease-fighting polyphenols. So, when we recommend coconut to you, we are *specifically* recommending "virgin" or "raw" coconut. Second, when you're following a low-carb diet, your body is better able to efficiently process coconut fat as an energy source.

New studies are constantly adding to the list of health benefits attributed to "virgin" and "raw" coconut products. For now, here's an abbreviated list: they are antioxidant and anti-inflammatory and they protect against infection, improve gut health, increase HDL, decrease blood triglycerides, and even increase fat burning. Indeed, human studies show that coconut oil's main fat, lauric acid, is burned more quickly than other fats. Lauric acid itself can also activate fat-burning proteins (nerd note: in particular, those in the PPAR family of transcription factors), just like oleic acid (see EVOO and avocado on pages 15 and 17) and palmitoleic acid (see macadamia nuts on page 19).

But the main reason we include coconut in this high-fat, low-carb New Mediterranean Diet comes down to what we call the fatome (an -ome term, similar to "genome" or "microbiome"), which is used to describe the complex mixture of fats you consume in your diet. Just as genes interact in your genome and microbes interact in your gut ecosystem, fats interact in your diet to collectively influence your health. In four simple words: *You Want Fatome Balance.* Early pre-published clinical observations suggest that, for people who follow a high-fat, low-carb Mediterranean diet, consuming some virgin or raw coconut may complement the fats found in the other six high-fat superfoods described above. Coconut may decrease your oxidizable fat load and contribute different antioxidants to your diet, improving your overall Fatome balance.

 PRACTICAL TIP

Only buy virgin or raw coconut products!

 KEY POINTS

① Although coconut is rich in saturated fat, the saturated fat is unique. Most of it doesn't go straight into your main blood circulation, but to your liver.

② Virgin or raw coconut is full of powerful antioxidants that fight disease.

③ Coconut harmonizes with the other high-fat superfoods described in this section, rounding out your fatome, and maybe slimming you out in the process, if that's your personal goal.

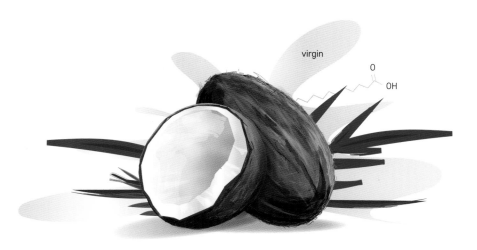

virgin

The Seven New Mediterranean High-Fat Superfoods!

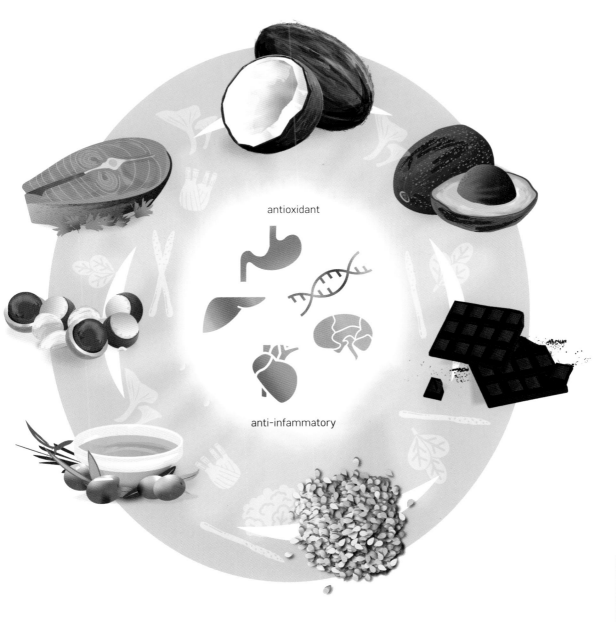

antioxidant

anti-infammatory

FOUR RUNNERS-UP

Although these foods aren't technically high-fat superfoods due to their lower fat content, they each deserve honorable mentions: chia seeds and flaxseeds, eggs, and liver.

① & ② Chia Seeds and Flaxseeds

We'll discuss chia seeds and flaxseeds together, because they both have a strikingly high fiber content, low net carb content, excellent fat profile, and high micronutrient density. Chia and flax each deliver at least 4 grams of fiber for every single gram of net carbs, a ratio that simply can't be beat.

Unlike other seeds (which are high in inflammatory omega-6 fats), chia and flax are rich in anti-inflammatory omega-3 fats. Although the specific type of omega-3 fat found in plant sources (ALA) is not as nutritionally favorable as those found in marine sources (EPA and DHA), it has still been linked in some studies to a reduced risk of heart disease and stroke. Making chia and flax your seeds of choice will improve your omega-6/3 ratio and decrease inflammation.

Finally, chia and flax are packed with an alphabet soup of micronutrients, including calcium, copper, iron, magnesium, manganese, niacin, phosphorus, potassium, selenium, and thiamine.

 PRACTICAL TIP

Curcumin, a compound found in turmeric, increases the conversion of ALA (plant omega-3) into its superior EPA and DHA (marine) forms. So, when possible, have turmeric with your seeds by making Superseed Crackers (page 70), which are delicious with our 4:1 Hummus (page 73). (By the way, this turmeric ALA kitchen hack isn't just fruitless biohacking. Combining turmeric and ALA has been shown to increase DHA levels in rat brains and to improve anxiety!)

③ Eggs

Eggs contain everything needed to bring forth life. Not surprisingly, they're packed with nutrients. They also contain zero carbs and have a 1:1 ratio of healthy fat to protein. The never-ending controversy over whether eggs are good for you or not is rooted in a misunderstanding of dietary cholesterol. First and foremost, only about 20 percent of the cholesterol in your blood comes from your diet. Most of it actually comes from your liver. Plus, when you eat less cholesterol, your liver simply makes more to compensate, and vice versa. For that reason alone, your dietary cholesterol intake isn't as big a deal as it's often made out to be. Second, cholesterol is an important nutrient your body needs in order to make cell membranes, hormones (e.g., testosterone and estrogen), brain cells, and the bile acids you need to properly digest the nutrients in your low-carb diet! If you're still wary of the cholesterol in eggs, never fear, we have awesome tricks listed in tip 3!

PRACTICAL TIPS

① Buy pastured (this differs from pasteurized, which means heated) or organic free-range eggs. These eggs come from chickens fed a natural diet and have the best omega-6/3 ratio. Omega-rich eggs are also good.

② The same turmeric trick we shared for chia and flax applies to the ALA in eggs.

③ There are at least five ways to decrease cholesterol absorption from eggs, if that's what you want. (Know that we are of the opinion that there is no reason to decrease your intake of dietary cholesterol.) These are:

- Eat MUFAs. Yay EVOO, avocados, and macadamia!

- Eat omega-3s. Yay fatty fish!

- Eat plenty of fiber. Yay avocado and veggies!

- Eat plant phytosterols. Plant sterols mimic cholesterol in the gut and bump cholesterol to the back of the line for absorption. Basically, the more phytosterols you eat, the more cholesterol you excrete.

- Get enough vitamin D. Vitamin D, which you can take as a supplement or get from exposure to direct sunlight, increases levels of the rate-limiting enzyme (cholesterol 7α hydroxylase) needed to convert cholesterol into bile acids. That means sunlight and vitamin D can decrease your blood cholesterol levels and increase your ability to process the nutrients in your low-carb, high-fat Mediterranean meals!

④ Liver

Liver is the canonical nutrient-dense superfood! A 5-ounce (140 g) portion contains at least 100 percent of the Recommended Dietary Allowances (RDAs) for vitamins A and B_{12}, choline, copper, niacin, and riboflavin, and at least 50 percent of the RDAs for vitamins B_5 and B_6, folate, iron, phosphorus, selenium, and zinc. Notably, some of these nutrients (vitamins A, B_6, B_{12}, and iron) are found in their more bioavailable, or active, forms in liver (as opposed to plant-based sources).

If you can't stomach the idea of eating organ meat, 100 percent grass-fed beef is an alternative. While it's not quite the nutritional equivalent of liver, grass-fed beef still has an impressive resume. Like all beef, it's packed with vitamin B_{12}, iron, and zinc. In addition, the diet of natural grass on which the animal was fed boosts the beef's fat profile in multiple ways. As compared to grain-fed beef, grass-fed beef has a far superior omega-6/3 ratio and up to 500 percent more "conjugated linoleic acid" (a special fatty acid made by the gut bacteria of cows and other ruminants, which, some studies suggest, can reduce the risk of obesity, type II diabetes, cancer, and heart disease).

ELEVEN FOUNDATIONAL VEGGIES

When it comes to low-carb vegetables, most believe it really is best to *eat the rainbow* (No! Not Starburst!). Certain vegetables feature prominently in this book and deserve special acclaim for their nutritional profiles.

Arugula is a great source of vitamins A, C, and K_1, calcium, folate, magnesium, and potassium. It gets its characteristic peppery flavor from erucin, a compound that is anti-inflammatory and has been demonstrated to slow the growth of, or even kill breast, colon, liver, leukemia, lung, and prostate cancer cells.

Asparagus spears are shaped like the number 1; could that be because asparagus contains an excellent 1:1:1 ratio of net carbs, fiber, and protein? It's also among the best prebiotic foods (that is, it feeds the healthy bacteria in your gut), and is a great source of vitamin K_1.

Bell Pepper (Red) is sweeter than its younger sibling, the green bell pepper, which is less ripe. However, for the additional 1 gram of sugar per pepper, you not only get extra flavor, but also 70 percent more vitamin C. In fact, bell peppers are among the vegetables richest in vitamin C. Vitamin C boosts immune function, supports heart health, and increases the absorption of the non-heme iron found in vegetables. This is important because non-heme iron is usually less well absorbed than the heme iron found in animal protein.

Cauliflower is not only the king of keto versatility, able to pinch-hit in place of dozens of comfort foods, but is also a surprisingly rich source of vitamin C. One cauliflower contains as much vitamin C as eight oranges! And if the "C" in cauliflower doesn't stand for vitamin C, it could stand for choline (an important brain-supporting nutrient found in few vegetables apart from cauliflower) or cancer-fighting, because sulforaphane, a compound found in cauliflower, is presumed to help kill cancer cells.

Eggplant soaks up fat and flavor like a sponge, which makes it perfect for a diet rich in yummy, healthy oils and spices. What's more, eggplants get their vibrant color from nasunin, an antioxidant that protects the heart and whose levels actually increase when eggplants are cooked. Just remember to leave the skin on.

Fennel stands out for its sweet, licoricey flavor. That sweetness doesn't come from sugar, but from a compound called anethol, which our taste buds perceive as thirteen times sweeter than sugar. Anethol relaxes the smooth muscles of the gastrointestinal tract to promote healthy bowel function.

Mushrooms are such a diverse group of organisms that you'd need a library to document their positive health effects. Here are just a few: they're great prebiotics, they decrease inflammation, and they may even protect against cognitive decline. Eating mushrooms at least twice per week is associated with a 50 percent decreased likelihood of developing Alzheimer's disease.

Red onions are second only to **capers** as the densest source of quercetin, one of nature's most powerful antioxidants. Quercetin levels are highest in the outermost rings of the onion and the area closest to the root. And, although onions contain a moderate amount of carbs, just a little onion packs a whole lot of flavor.

Spinach is extremely low in carbs, with only 1 gram of net carbs per 100 grams. It's also a natural multivitamin, containing impressive amounts of vitamins A, C, K, folate, magnesium, and potassium. Plus, it cooks down well, allowing you to get an even greater density of nutrients in a single serving.

Watercress is remarkably low in calories, even for a leafy green vegetable, with only 11 calories per 100 grams. However, these measly 11 calories contain 60 to 70 percent of the RDAs for vitamins A and C, and 300 percent of the RDA for vitamin K_1. The similarity between the nutrition profiles of arugula and watercress is no coincidence; both belong to the same family of vegetables that includes **Brussels sprouts, broccoli, cabbage,** and **cauliflower**, or cruciferous vegetables. There is a great degree of nutritional overlap among cruciferous vegetables, and all are thought to be particularly good at preventing cancer because they contain anticancer glucosinolates, a family of cancer-killing compounds that includes our friends erucin (found in arugula) and sulforaphane (found in cauliflower).

Zucchini are surprisingly sweet, considering their low-carb profile, and contain more potassium than a banana. They get their green color from lutein and zeaxanthin, antioxidants that are great for eye health, protecting visual acuity against age. Plus, they pair particularly well with the flavors of EVOO, avocado, and macadamia, and can be spiralized into an excellent and fun-to-eat replacement for noodles.

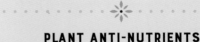

PLANT ANTI-NUTRIENTS

Within the nutrition science community there has recently been debate regarding the potentially harmful effects of certain plant "anti-nutrients." These compounds—including lectins, phytates, and oxalates—are thought to play potentially negative roles in health by preventing the absorption of essential minerals, contributing to leaky gut and chronic low-grade inflammation, and so on. We, the authors of *The New Mediterranean Diet Cookbook*, are currently of the opinion that such claims are backed by the scientific literature and that some people do benefit from the reduction or elimination of these anti-nutrients. However, as not all people appear to be equally sensitive to all anti-nutrients, it's important for you, dear reader, to weigh for yourself the relative pros and cons of foods containing these compounds to decide whether you think you should include them as part of your diet.

UNDERSTANDING RECIPE NUTRITION

Each recipe in this book comes with a basic macronutrient breakdown, including total grams of net carbs, fiber, protein, and fat. Also included are percentages, corresponding to the proportion of calories each macronutrient contributes to the dish.

Because standard ketogenic diets contain less than 5 to 10 percent calories from carbs, we keep net carbs below 10 percent for all recipes in this book, except for some sides and basics, which are intended to be consumed as part of complete meals that contain less than 10 percent of overall calories from carbs.

But we're sure you've seen basic macronutrient breakdowns before. They're not terribly exciting.

What's truly exciting about this book is that it's the first to include a proper *Fat Profile!* We feel this is important because sustainable low-carb diets are necessarily high in fats, and not all fats are created equal. Far from it! (Remember the fish tails metaphor in the discussion of fatty acids on page 12?)

The first component of a recipe's Fat Profile is the **SAT/MUFA/PUFA** breakdown: the percentage of fat in a recipe that is saturated, monounsaturated, or polyunsaturated.

As a guideline, you want high MUFA, lower PUFA, and saturated fats to fill in the rest.

The second component is the **omega-6/3 ratio**.

As a guideline, you want a lower omega-6/3 ratio.

Pretty simple so far. However, there are important nuances to these guidelines. Here's a list of things to consider.

- There is usually a **compromise between MUFA and omega-6/3**. This is because high-MUFA sources often contain a reasonable amount of omega-6 (avocado oil, for example, contains around 14 percent), and low-omega-6 sources are usually richer in saturated fats, as opposed to MUFA (for example, ghee). In the end, you probably want a nice balance between MUFA and your omega-6/3 ratio.

  We're drawing particular attention to the examples of high-MUFA **avocado oil** and low-omega-6 **ghee** because they are the two staple cooking fats we use in this book. In general, they are interchangeable, and you should choose which one to use based on whether you want to push up your MUFA intake or decrease your omega-6 intake at any given time.

  As an aside, **macadamia oil** has a high smoke point and is high–MUFA (80 percent) and extremely low in omega-6 (2 percent). Therefore, macadamia oil allows you to avoid the compromise between high MUFA and low omega-6. However, it's more expensive, and therefore simply isn't a practical choice for most people.

- You'll notice that, in some recipes, we report an omega-6/3 ratio, while in others, we report only omega-6 levels in grams. This is because not all fat sources contain omega-3s, but most contain some omega-6. Therefore, if a dish lacks an omega-3 source (which is okay—you don't need omega-3 at every meal), the ratio would give an unfairly negative representation of the recipe's fat profile.

  More to the point, your overall dietary omega-6/3 ratio is determined by the omega-6/3 ratio in omega-3-rich meals combined with the absolute omega-6 contents of your lower omega-3 meals.

- It's important to note that the omega-6 in whole foods are not the same as the toxic omega-6 found in industrially produced, processed vegetable oils. Nature and evolution have packaged whole foods to be way healthier!

For example, remember how tahini breaks the "omega-6 is bad" rule because it features the Terrific Trio of lignan antioxidants (page 22)? Well, the same principle applies to other whole foods.

By contrast, the omega-6 you might consume when you eat processed foods have been isolated, separated from their natural nutritional partners, and otherwise corrupted and damaged by heat or toxic chemical exposures. But you won't have to worry about that when you make the recipes in this book. All of our recipes use only whole foods, preferably bought raw.

So, to sum up, when cooking at high temperatures, choose avocado oil to push up your MUFAs or ghee to decrease your omega-6/3 ratio. The choice is yours, and it depends on your priorities and nutritional perspective. Macadamia oil optimizes both, but again, it's more expensive.

When a dish doesn't have an omega-3 source, we instead report the absolute amount of omega-6, because that information is more useful.

And, of course, simply eating whole foods that are packaged in the way nature intended means you're way ahead of where you'd be nutritionally if you were eating processed foods.

NOTE

Nutrition values for each recipe in this book are per serving unless stated otherwise. The nutrition data are derived from the USDA National Nutrient Database (ndb.nal.usda.gov). Peer-reviewed data from PubMed Central National Center for Biotechnology Information (pubmed.ncbi.nlm.nih.gov) were also used to supplement pieces of data absent on the USDA database for particular foods. Nutrition facts are calculated from edible parts. For example, if one large avocado is listed as 7 ounces (200 g), this value represents its edible parts (pit and peel removed) unless otherwise specified. Similarly, if one fennel bulb is listed as 14.1 ounces (400 g), this value excludes hard fennel stems that are discarded before preparing the recipe.

Recipes that include pesto use Macadamia Basil Pesto (page 198) for the nutritional calculations, unless otherwise specified.

Blanched almond flour, which is made from blanched almonds, is preferable to almond meal, which is made from whole almonds. Hazelnut flour is better still, as it's higher in MUFA and lower in omega-6.

No recipes in this book require sweeteners. However, optional low-carb approved sweeteners, such as stevia or erythritol, can be used in some recipes. But be warned: While stevia and erythritol are largely non-insulinogenic and usually well tolerated, individuals prone to gastrointestinal distress (including conditions such as IBS or SIBO) may want to avoid any and all sweeteners because of their potential impact on symptoms.

OTHER INGREDIENTS USED IN THIS BOOK

Avocado: preferably Hass/California

Fats: virgin, cold-pressed avocado oil, macadamia oil and coconut oil; 100% grass-fed ghee; extra-virgin olive oil (See the Superfoods section for shopping tips.)

Vegetables to purchase organic: bell peppers, tomatoes, spinach, and other leafy greens. Not all vegetables need to be labeled organic to be safe to eat. To find an up-to-date list of which vegetables you should always buy organic, check out the Dirty Dozen list (www.ewg.org).

Meat: 100% grass-fed lamb, beef, and liver. Pork: outdoor reared and organic. Chicken and eggs: pastured (U.S.), or organic, free-range (U.K.), no corn or soy or antibiotics

Dairy: dairy products from sheep's or goat's milk, such as cream, feta, Manchego, and Pecorino; mozzarella from buffalo's milk

Fish: wild salmon, ideally wild Alaskan sockeye; tuna, ideally light or skipjack tuna; canned fish, such as sardines, in brine or water. Avoid farmed fish, too, and choose wild-caught, locally sourced, sustainable fish that's low in mercury. For more information, visit www.seafoodwatch.org.

Coconut, nuts, and seeds: raw and unsalted

Other ingredients: pink Himalayan salt, Ceylon cinnamon, cacao (rather than cocoa), or high-flavanol chocolate

RECIPE ICONS

All recipes are tagged with these icons, as needed. Here are the tags you will find in our recipes:

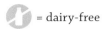 = dairy-free

 = egg-free

 = nut-free

= nightshade-free

= vegetarian

Recipes that include gray versions of the icons meet the criteria for the regular icons, but only if you use provided alternate ingredients or omit certain toppings or suggested sides.

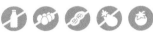

In the nutritional facts, the ☺ icon is used in cases when the ratio is less than or equal to 2.0 to positively emphasize the fact that the reccipe has a particularly excellent ratio of omegas 6 and 3.

AN IMPORTANT NOTE ABOUT MEASUREMENTS

It's best to use a kitchen scale to measure ingredients—using cups or tablespoons can lead to inaccuracies that may affect the finished product, especially with dry ingredients used in baked goods.

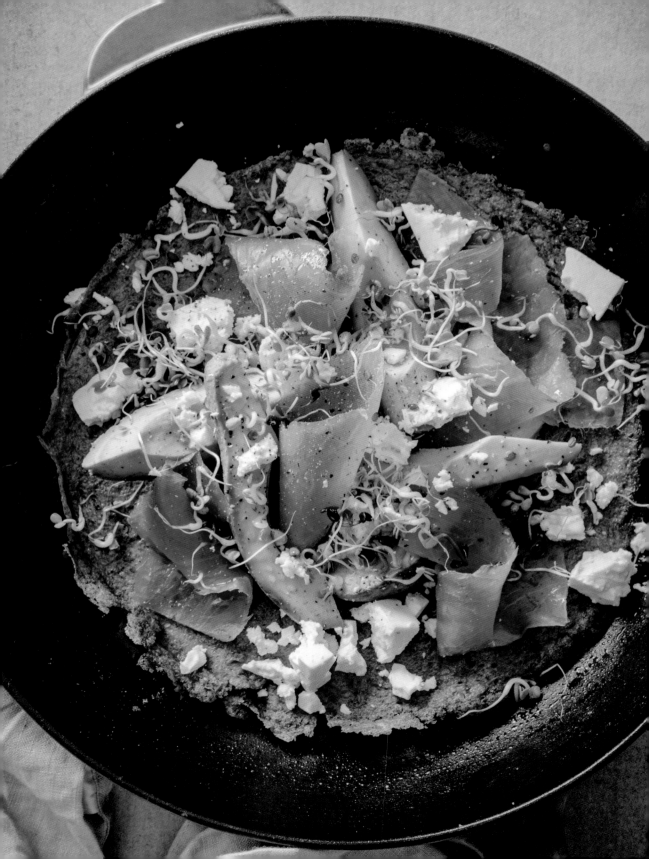

CHAPTER 2

BREAKFASTS

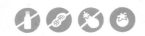

SUPERFOOD OMELET, TWO WAYS

Omelets are *the* go-to breakfast for people who appreciate simplicity. Just like an egg yolk contains all the foundational nutrients required to nurture a new life, omelets can set you up for the day practically every day, because they're incredibly versatile. These Turkish- and Greek-inspired vegetarian versions are just two pieces of proof that the trusty omelet is anything but boring.

TURKISH-STYLE FILLING

1 tablespoon (15 ml) extra-virgin avocado oil or ghee

¼ small (15 g/0.5 oz) red onion, sliced

½ medium (60 g/2.1 oz) red bell pepper, sliced

4 to 6 leaves (30 g/1.1 oz) cavolo nero or curly kale, stems removed and torn into pieces or chopped

1 medium (85 g/3 oz) tomato, chopped

½ teaspoon ground cumin

Salt and black pepper, to taste

1 tablespoon (4 g/0.2 oz) chopped fresh parsley or cilantro

GREEK-STYLE FILLING

1 tablespoon (15 ml) extra-virgin avocado oil or ghee

3 cups (90 g/3.2 oz) fresh spinach

½ teaspoon dried oregano

4 to 6 leaves fresh mint, chopped

Salt and black pepper, to taste if needed

6 pitted Kalamata olives (18 g/0.6 oz), sliced

¼ cup (35 g/1.2 oz) crumbled feta cheese

2 teaspoons (10 ml) extra-virgin olive oil, to drizzle

OMELET

2 teaspoons (10 ml) extra-virgin avocado oil or ghee

2 large eggs

1 egg yolk

¼ teaspoon ground turmeric

Pinch of salt and black pepper

① To make the Turkish-style filling: Grease a large skillet with the avocado oil. Add the onion and cook for 3 to 5 minutes, until fragrant. Add the bell pepper and cavolo nero and cook for 2 to 3 minutes. Add the tomato, cumin, salt, pepper, and parsley, and mix well. Transfer to a bowl and set aside while you prepare the omelet.

② To make the Greek-style filling: Grease a large skillet with the avocado oil. Add the spinach and cook for about 1 minute, until wilted. Add the oregano, mint, salt, and pepper, and mix well. Transfer to a bowl, and add the olives, feta, and olive oil. Set aside while you prepare the omelet.

③ To make the omelet: Heat a large skillet greased with the avocado oil over medium heat. Whisk the eggs with the yolk, then add the turmeric, salt, and pepper. Pour the eggs into the pan and cook, lifting the edges with a spatula and tilting the pan to allow uncooked egg to run under the omelet. When the omelet is almost done but still moist on top, spread the topping of choice across the top of the omelet. Gently fold in half and cook for 1 to 2 minutes, until cooked through. Eat immediately or store in the fridge for up to 1 day.

NUTRITION FACTS PER SERVING (1 TURKISH/GREEK OMELET):

Total carbs: 12.1/8.2 g	Fat: 38.2/59.1 g (of which saturated: 7.5/15.3 g)	Saturated / MUFA / PUFA (%): 20, 68, 12 / 26, 64, 10
Fiber: 3.9/3.3 g	Calories: 459/652 kcal	Omega-6/3 ratio: 3.4/3.8
Net Carbs: 8.2/4.9 g	Macronutrient ratio: Calories from carbs (7/3%), protein (16/15%), fat (77/82%)	
Protein: 18.2/23.7 g		

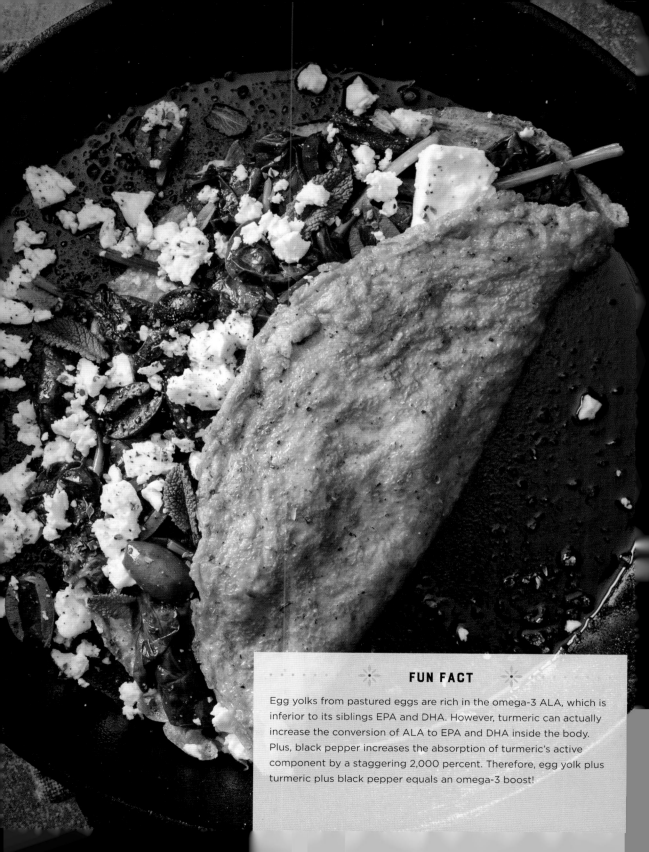

FUN FACT

Egg yolks from pastured eggs are rich in the omega-3 ALA, which is inferior to its siblings EPA and DHA. However, turmeric can actually increase the conversion of ALA to EPA and DHA inside the body. Plus, black pepper increases the absorption of turmeric's active component by a staggering 2,000 percent. Therefore, egg yolk plus turmeric plus black pepper equals an omega-3 boost!

QUICK LOW-CARB AVOCADO TOASTS

These easy-to-make, open-faced sandwiches are made with keto-friendly "bread" you can whip up in the microwave. Make a double batch of the base in advance, then pair with your favorite toppings for an I'm-already-late-for-work breakfast. We use smashed avocado here, but you can also try Cod Liver & Egg Salad (page 92), smoked salmon, or sardines and goat's cheese.

QUICK BREAD BASE

¼ cup (28 g/1 oz) flax meal

2 tablespoons (16 g/0.6 oz) coconut flour

2 teaspoons (2 g) psyllium powder

⅛ teaspoon baking soda

Optional: ½ teaspoon dried herbs, ¼ teaspoon paprika or ground turmeric

Salt and black pepper, to taste

¼ teaspoon apple cider vinegar

1 teaspoon extra-virgin olive oil or ghee, plus more for greasing

1 large egg

2 tablespoons (30 ml) water

AVOCADO TOPPING

1 large (200 g/7 oz) ripe avocado

¼ small (15 g/0.5 oz) red onion or 1 spring onion, minced

1 tablespoon (15 ml) extra-virgin olive oil

1 tablespoon (15 ml) fresh lemon juice

Salt, black pepper, and/or chile flakes, to taste

2 teaspoons (2–3 g) chopped fresh herbs, such as parsley or chives

Optional: 2 ounces (57 g) smoked salmon and/or poached egg

① To make the bread base: Combine all the dry ingredients in a bowl. Add the wet ingredients. Combine and set aside for 5 minutes. Divide the mixture between two wide ramekins lightly greased with the olive oil and microwave on high for about 2 minutes, checking every 30 to 60 seconds to avoid overcooking. (If the bread ends up too dry, you can "rehydrate" it: Pour 1 tablespoon [15 ml] of water evenly over it, then return it to the microwave for 30 seconds.) Let it cool slightly, then cut widthwise. Place on a dry non-stick pan and toast for 1 to 2 minutes per side. Set aside.

② To make the topping: In a bowl, mash the avocado with the onion, oil, lemon juice, salt, pepper, and chile flakes. To serve, spread the avocado mixture on top of the sliced bread and add fresh herbs. Optionally, top with smoked salmon. Store the bread separately from the topping at room temperature in a sealed container for 1 day, in the fridge for up to 5 days, or freeze for up to 3 months. Refrigerate the topping in a sealed jar for up to 3 days.

 FUN FACT

When avocados ripen, the enzyme phenylalanine ammonia-lyase makes polyphenols. In brief, ripe avocados are healthier!

NUTRITION FACTS PER SERVING (2 TOASTS):

Total carbs: 18.4 g	Fat: 31 g (of which saturated: 5.5 g)	Without Salmon:
Fiber: 14.1 g	Calories: 367 kcal	Saturated / MUFA / PUFA (%): 18, 61, 21
Net Carbs: 4.3 g	Macronutrient ratio: Calories from carbs (5%), protein (11%), fat (84%)	Omega-6/3 ratio: 1.0 ☺
Protein: 9.4 g		

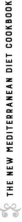

GREEN SPINACH & SALMON CREPES

(CONTRIBUTOR: EMILY MAGUIRE)

These green and grain-free keto crepes are courtesy of Emily Maguire, a certified nutritionist with an additional degree in Obesity Science who spends her time traveling the world lecturing to scientists about the benefits of ketogenic diets. With a decade of experience helping people lose weight on low-carb, she knows what works. "Blending spinach into the batter gives these crepes a lovely vibrant color and extra vitamins. A little nutritional yeast boosts B vitamins and adds a bold, cheesy flavor. Paired with omega-3-rich wild salmon and MUFA-rich avocado, they make an elegant and healthy weekend breakfast."

GREEN SPINACH CREPE

1 cup (30 g/1.1 oz) fresh spinach or thawed and drained frozen spinach

1 small bunch (8 g/0.3 oz) fresh parsley

½ teaspoon fresh thyme leaves or ¼ teaspoon dried thyme

1 tablespoon (12 g/0.4 oz) nutritional yeast

1 tablespoon (7 g/0.3 oz) flax meal

Salt and black pepper, to taste

2 large eggs

2 teaspoons (10 ml) extra-virgin avocado oil or ghee for cooking

SALMON FILLING

3 ounces (85 g) wild smoked salmon

½ large (100 g/3.5 oz) avocado, sliced

2 tablespoons (20 g/0.7 oz) crumbled goat's cheese or feta

1 teaspoon fresh lemon or lime juice

Optional: fresh herbs or microgreens, to taste

① To make the green spinach crepe: Place the spinach, herbs, nutritional yeast, flax meal, salt, and pepper in a food processor or blender. Process well until the spinach is finely chopped. Add the eggs and process on low speed until the mixture is just combined.

② Heat half of the oil in a large skillet and add half of the mixture. Swirl the pan so the mixture completely covers the bottom. Cook for about 3 minutes or until just set, then add the salmon and avocado. Sprinkle the crepe with the goat's cheese and drizzle with the lemon juice. Slide onto a plate and optionally garnish with fresh herbs or microgreens. Serve warm.

 FUN FACT

This breakfast is fructose-free. Eating too much fructose can overwhelm the small intestine, toxify the liver, and increase de novo lipogenesis, which is when your body turns carbs into fat that gets stored as body fat!

NUTRITION FACTS PER SERVING (1 CREPE):

Total carbs: 19.3 g	Fat: 49.2 g (of which saturated: 11.6 g)	Saturated / MUFA / PUFA (%): 24, 61, 15
Fiber: 12.7 g	Calories: 679 kcal	Omega-6/3 ratio: 1.0 ☺
Net Carbs: 6.6 g	Macronutrient ratio: Calories from carbs (4%), protein (27%), fat (69%)	
Protein: 44.4 g		

BREAKFASTS

GREEK BREAKFAST POWER BOWL

Full of protein, antioxidant-rich veggies, and healthy fats, this Mediterranean-inspired all-day breakfast bowl will keep you satisfied until lunchtime and beyond. Tender, low-carb, herb-enhanced veggies are topped with soft-boiled eggs and addictively salty Halloumi and olives, plus a final flourish of extra-virgin olive oil for an added dose of disease-fighting oleic acid.

3 tablespoons (45 ml) extra-virgin avocado oil or ghee, divided

1 clove garlic, minced

2 teaspoons (2 g) chopped fresh rosemary

1 small (200 g/7 oz) eggplant, roughly chopped

1 medium (200 g/7 oz) zucchini, roughly chopped

1 tablespoon (15 ml) fresh lemon juice

2 tablespoons (6 g/0.2 oz) chopped mint

1 tablespoon (3 g/0.1 oz) chopped fresh oregano

Salt and black pepper, to taste

6 ounces (170 g) Halloumi cheese, cubed or sliced

¼ cup (25 g/0.9 oz) pitted Kalamata olives

4 large eggs, soft-boiled (or hard-boiled or poached)

1 tablespoon (15 ml) extra-virgin olive oil, to drizzle

① Heat a skillet (with a lid) greased with 2 tablespoons (30 ml) of the avocado oil over medium heat. Add the garlic and rosemary and cook for 1 minute. Add the eggplant, zucchini, and lemon juice. Stir and cover with a lid, then reduce the heat to medium-low. Cook for 10 to 15 minutes, stirring once or twice, until tender.

② Stir in the mint and oregano. Optionally, reserve some herbs for topping. Season with salt and pepper to taste. Remove from the heat and transfer to a plate. Cover with the skillet lid to keep the veggies warm.

③ Grease the same pan with the remaining 1 tablespoon (15 ml) avocado oil and cook the Halloumi over medium-high heat for 2 to 3 minutes per side until lightly browned. Place the slices of cooked Halloumi on top of the cooked veggies. Top with the olives and cooked eggs and drizzle with the olive oil.

④ Always serve warm, as Halloumi hardens once it cools. Reheat before serving if necessary.

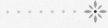

FUN FACT

Oleic acid in the olives, olive oil, and avocado oil in this dish has been shown to protect GLP-1 secreting L-cells in the gut. This is good because GLP-1 crosses into the brain and helps with synaptic plasticity. More synaptic plasticity means more connections among your brain cells, which protects against cognitive decline.

NUTRITION FACTS PER SERVING (1 BOWL):

Total carbs: 13.8 g	Fat: 58 g (of which saturated: 17.9 g)	Saturated / MUFA / PUFA (%): 31, 59, 10
Fiber: 5.2 g	Calories: 679 kcal	Omega-6/3 ratio: 3.6
Net Carbs: 8.6 g	Macronutrient ratio: Calories from carbs (5%), protein (17%), fat (78%)	
Protein: 27.7 g		

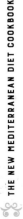

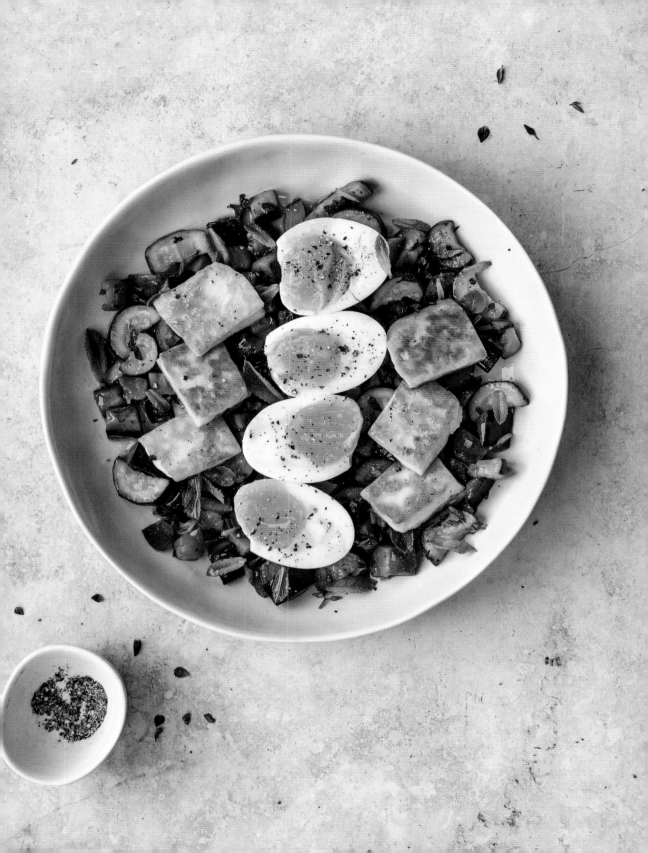

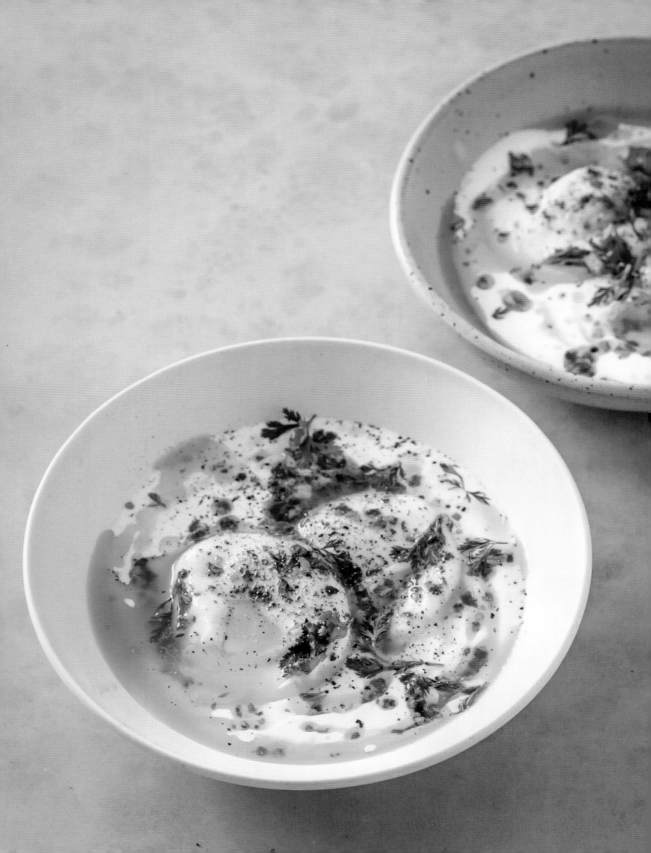

TURKISH EGG BOWL

This is vegetarian comfort food at its best, and it's such an innovative way to serve breakfast eggs—with healthy fats, fresh herbs, and a spicy chile kick. If you've never had goat's milk yogurt before, you're in for a treat! Like goat's cheese, a staple of Turkish cuisine, its flavor is wonderfully grassy and earthy. Plus, goat and sheep dairy products are free of the pro-inflammatory A1 casein found in cow's milk, and also contain smaller fat droplets that are easier to digest.

2 tablespoons (30 ml) ghee

½–1 teaspoon red chile flakes

2 tablespoons (30 ml) extra-virgin olive oil

1 cup (250 g/8.8 oz) full-fat goat's or sheep's milk yogurt

1 clove garlic, minced

1 tablespoon (15 ml) fresh lemon juice

Salt and black pepper, to taste

Dash of vinegar

4 large eggs

Optional: pinch of sumac

2 tablespoons (8 g/0.3 oz) chopped fresh cilantro or parsley

① In a skillet, melt the ghee over low heat. Add the chile flakes and let it infuse while you prepare the eggs. Remove from the heat and mix with the extra-virgin olive oil. Set aside. Combine the yogurt, garlic, lemon juice, salt, and pepper.

② Poach the eggs. Fill a medium saucepan with water and a dash of vinegar. Bring to a boil over high heat. Crack each egg individually into a ramekin or a cup. Using a spoon, create a gentle whirlpool in the water; this will help the egg white wrap around the egg yolk. Slowly lower the egg into the water in the center of the whirlpool. Turn off the heat and cook for 3 to 4 minutes. Use a slotted spoon to remove the egg from the water and place it on a plate. Repeat for all remaining eggs.

③ To assemble, place the yogurt mixture in a bowl and add the poached eggs. Drizzle with the infused oil, and garnish with cilantro. Add a pinch of sumac, if using. Eat warm.

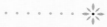 **FUN FACT**

The American Institute of Medicine and the Food Nutrition Board acknowledged that carbohydrates are a nonessential dietary nutrient and that life requires zero carbohydrates in the diet.

NUTRITION FACTS PER SERVING (1 BOWL):

Total carbs: 8.2 g

Fiber: 0.8 g

Net Carbs: 7.4 g

Protein: 21.9 g

Fat: 47.4 g (of which saturated: 20.3 g)

Calories: 542 kcal

Macronutrient ratio: Calories from carbs (5%), protein (16%), fat (79%)

Saturated / MUFA / PUFA (%): 43, 50, 7

Omega-6/3 ratio: 2.5

GOLDEN EGG SKILLET

These easy skillet eggs are lovely to look at, but trust us, they're not just a pretty face. Paired with low-carb veggies such as zucchini and chard and laced with turmeric, our Golden Egg Skillet packs enormous anti-inflammatory benefits. Don't even think about skipping the black pepper: it significantly improves the body's absorption of curcumin, turmeric's active component.

2 tablespoons (30 ml) extra-virgin avocado oil or ghee

2 medium (30 g/1.1 oz) spring onions, white and green parts separated, sliced

1 clove garlic, minced

3.5 ounces (100 g) Swiss chard or collard greens, stalks and leaves separated, chopped

1 medium (200 g/7 oz) zucchini, sliced into coins

2 tablespoons (30 ml) water

1 teaspoon Dijon or yellow mustard

½ teaspoon ground turmeric

¼ teaspoon black pepper

Salt, to taste

4 large eggs

¾ cup (85 g/3 oz) grated Manchego or Pecorino Romano cheese

2 tablespoons (30 ml) extra-virgin olive oil

① Preheat the oven to 360°F (180°C) fan assisted or 400°F (200°C) conventional.

② Grease a large, ovenproof skillet (with a lid) with the avocado oil. Cook the white parts of the spring onions and the garlic for about 1 minute, until just fragrant. Add the chard stalks, zucchini, and water. Stir, then cover with a lid. Cook over medium-low heat for about 10 minutes or until the zucchini is tender. Add the mustard, turmeric, pepper, and salt. Add the chard leaves and cook until just wilted.

③ Use a spatula to make 4 wells in the mixture. Crack an egg into each well and cook until the egg whites start to set while the yolks are still runny. Top with the cheese, transfer to the oven, and bake for 5 to 7 minutes. Remove from the oven and sprinkle with the reserved spring onions. Drizzle with the olive oil and serve warm.

 FUN FACT

Harder and less acidic cheeses are typically higher in calcium, in part because the lactic acid produced by bacteria during the fermentation process in cheese making dissolves calcium. Manchego is far richer in calcium than Brie or blue cheeses.

NUTRITION FACTS PER SERVING:

Total carbs: 8.1 g	Fat: 48.2 g (of which saturated: 14.4 g)	Saturated / MUFA / PUFA (%): 30, 61, 9
Fiber: 2.5 g	Calories: 560 kcal	Omega-6: 3.8 g
Net Carbs: 5.6 g	Macronutrient ratio: Calories from carbs (4%), protein (18%), fat (78%)	
Protein: 25.9 g		

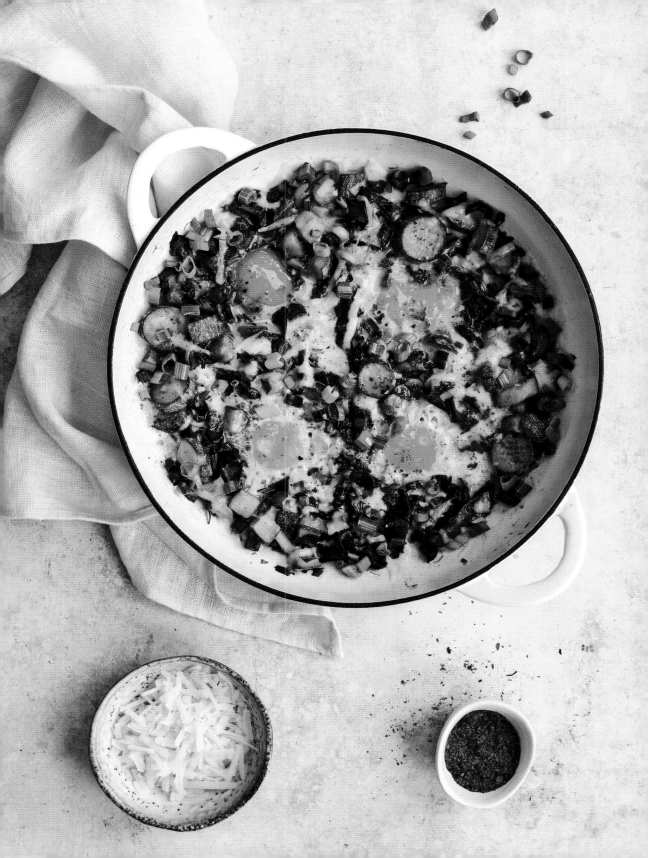

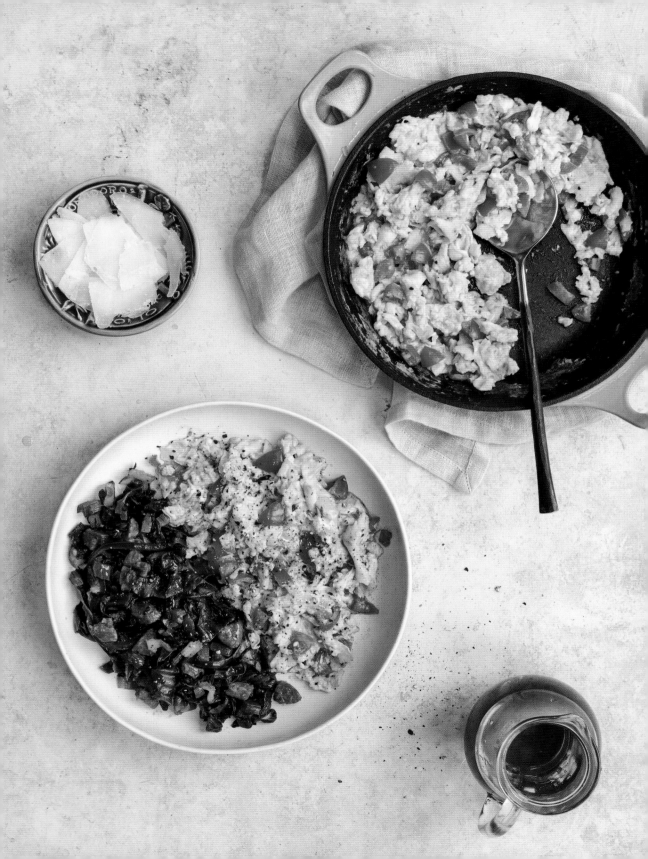

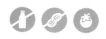

SPANISH SCRAMBLE

Scrambled eggs make a simple and satisfying keto breakfast all on their own, but adding spicy, oily chorizo really makes them sing. Here, they're paired with juicy tomatoes and crunchy chard and a handful of Manchego cheese for a well-balanced meal that features plenty of healthy fats.

CHORIZO & CHARD

1 tablespoon (15 ml) extra-virgin avocado oil or ghee

½ small (30 g/1.1 oz) red onion, sliced

7 ounces (200 g) chard, leaves and stalks separated, chopped

3 ounces (85 g) Mexican chorizo

SCRAMBLED EGGS

4 large eggs

2 egg yolks

Salt and black pepper, to taste

1 tablespoon (15 ml) extra-virgin avocado oil or ghee

3 ounces (85 g) cherry tomatoes or regular tomatoes, diced

1 tablespoon (15 ml) extra-virgin olive oil

Optional: 2 ounces (57 g) shaved Manchego cheese and chopped fresh herbs of choice, such as basil or parsley

① To make the chorizo & chard: Heat a skillet greased with the avocado oil. Add the sliced onion and cook for 2 to 3 minutes, until fragrant. Add the chard stalks and chorizo and cook for 5 to 8 minutes, until cooked through. Add the chard leaves and cook until just wilted. Remove from the heat and transfer to a plate.

② To make the scrambled eggs: In a bowl, whisk the eggs and egg yolks with a pinch of salt and pepper. Grease the same skillet in which you cooked the chorizo with the avocado oil. Pour in the eggs and swirl the pan to coat the bottom. Using a rubber spatula, gently push the edges into the middle of the pan. The uncooked runny eggs should spill out and coat the base of the pan.

③ After about 1 minute, add the tomatoes. Cook until the eggs are just set, then remove from the heat. Drizzle the eggs with the olive oil and optionally add the Manchego cheese and chopped herbs. Serve warm with the cooked chorizo and chard.

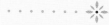

FUN FACT

Manchego is sheep's cheese and therefore "A2." Consumption of A1 dairy from cows, however, is associated with increased prevalence of autoimmune diseases, like type I diabetes.

NUTRITION FACTS PER SERVING:

Total carbs: 9.2 g	Fat: 43.5 g (of which saturated: 7.3 g)	Saturated / MUFA / PUFA (%): 17, 72, 11
Fiber: 2.8 g	Calories: 522 kcal	Omega-6/3 ratio: 3.6
Net Carbs: 6.4 g	Macronutrient ratio: Calories from carbs	
Protein: 24.4 g	(5%), protein (19%), fat (76%)	

SUPERFOOD SHAKSHUKA

(CONTRIBUTOR: DR. MARK CUCUZZELLA)

Shakshuka is a Mediterranean breakfast dish in which eggs are gently baked in a tomato-based sauce, and lately it's been popping up on brunch menus just about everywhere. This avocado-topped version was contributed by Dr. Mark Cucuzzella, a physician, author, father, professor of medicine, and superstar runner who has completed more than a hundred marathons and ultramarathons and who knows a thing or two about how diet affects sports performance. Mark says, "For me, eggs, sheep's and goat's cheese, and colorful non-starchy vegetables are magic foods. By preventing inflammation, they help my body burn clean!"

SKILLET

2 tablespoons (30 ml) extra-virgin avocado oil or ghee

½ small (30 g/1.1 oz) red onion, chopped

1 clove garlic, minced

1 small (85 g/3 oz) green bell pepper, sliced

1 small (150 g/5.3 oz) zucchini, chopped

½ teaspoon ground cumin

½ teaspoon ground turmeric

¼ teaspoon ground coriander

½ teaspoon paprika

3.5 ounces (100 g) spinach, fresh or frozen, thawed and drained

½ cup (120 ml) canned chopped or whole tomatoes

4 large eggs

TOPPINGS

1 small (100 g/3.5 oz) avocado, sliced

2 teaspoons (10 ml) fresh lemon juice

¼ cup (37 g/1.3 oz) crumbled feta or goat's cheese

2 tablespoons (30 ml) extra-virgin olive oil

① Preheat the oven to 400°F (200°C) fan assisted or 425°F (220°C) conventional.

② To make the skillet: Heat the oil in a large, ovenproof skillet over medium-high heat. Add the onion, garlic, bell pepper, and zucchini. Sauté for 3 to 4 minutes until soft. Add the spices and cook for 30 seconds until fragrant, then add the spinach and tomatoes. Cook until the spinach is wilted, about 1 minute. Turn off the heat.

③ Using a spoon, create 4 wells in the sauce and crack an egg into each well. Transfer the skillet to the oven and cook for 5 to 8 minutes just until the egg whites are set but the yolks are still runny.

④ Top with the avocado, lemon juice, feta, and olive oil. Serve immediately.

 FUN FACT

Once you fat-adapt your body to a high-fat, low-carb diet, it can burn twice as much fat during exercise than it could before.

NUTRITION FACTS PER SERVING:

Total carbs: 17.1 g	Fat: 49.3 g (of which saturated: 10.7 g)	Saturated / MUFA / PUFA (%): 22, 67, 11
Fiber: 7.9 g	Calories: 573 kcal	Omega-6/3 ratio: 4.4
Net Carbs: 9.2 g	Macronutrient ratio: Calories from carbs (7%), protein (14%), fat (79%)	
Protein: 20 g		

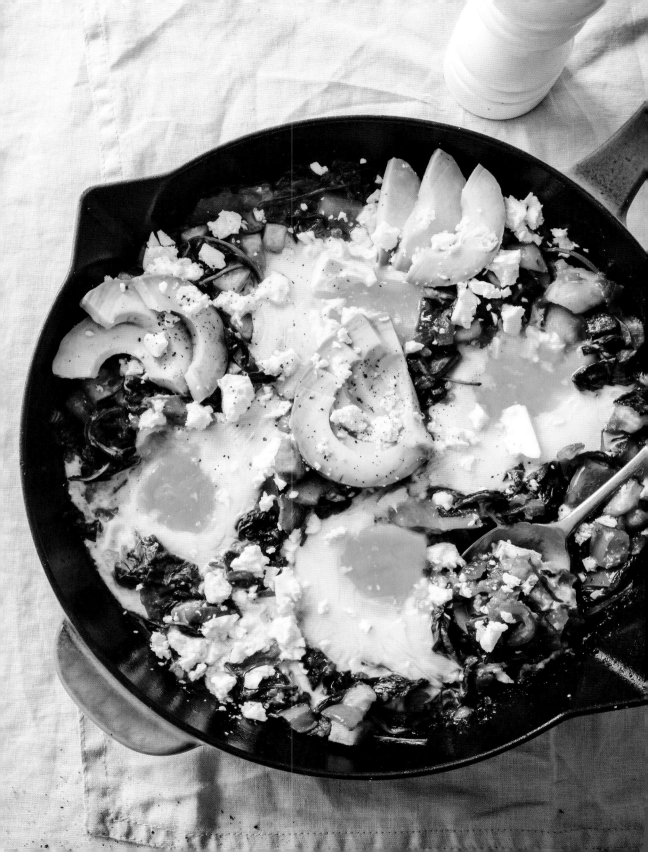

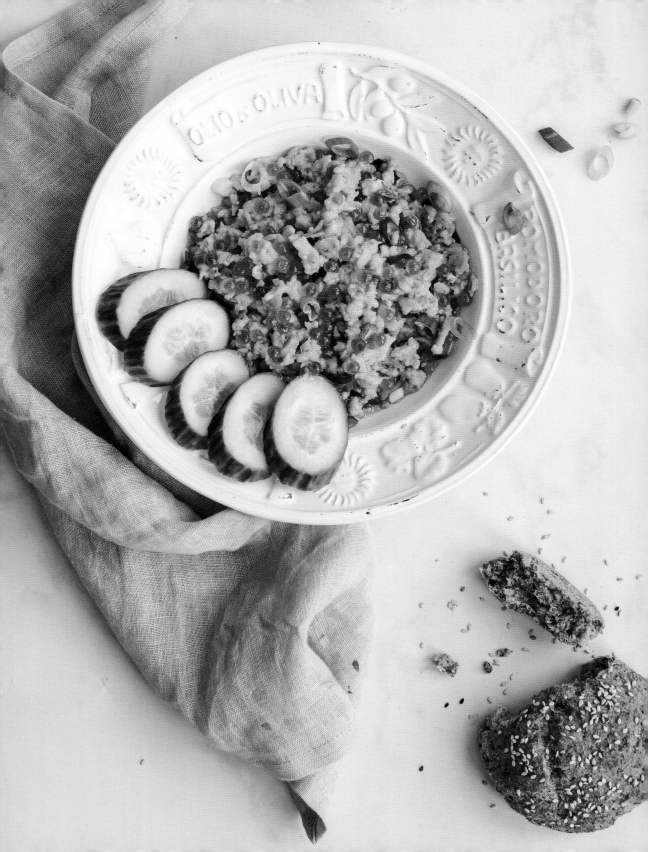

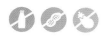

SALMON ROE & EGG CRUSH

Eggs from both the land and the sea: it's a breakfast surf and turf! By now you know that eggs are among the healthiest foods on the planet, because they contain everything needed to support a new life. Here's even better news: salmon eggs are the world's best source of omega-3! Made with just a few simple ingredients, this luxuriously creamy dish is delicious with a side of veggies and a slice of Quick Low-Carb Bread, (page 38).

3 large eggs

1 large egg yolk

¼ teaspoon ground turmeric

Optional: ¼ cup (15 g/0.5 oz) grated Pecorino Romano

1 tablespoon (15 ml) ghee or extra-virgin avocado oil

1 medium spring onion, white and green parts separated, sliced

Salt and black pepper, to taste

1 tablespoon (15 ml) extra-virgin olive oil

¼ cup (50 g/1.8 oz) salmon roe

Optional: sliced vegetables and Quick Low-Carb Bread (page 38), to serve

① In a bowl, whisk together the eggs, egg yolk, turmeric, and optionally the grated cheese.

② Grease a skillet with the ghee. Add the white parts of the spring onion and cook over medium heat for 2 to 3 minutes, until fragrant.

③ Pour in the egg mixture and swirl the pan to coat the bottom. Sprinkle with salt and pepper. Using a rubber spatula, gently push the edges into the middle of the pan. The uncooked runny eggs should spill out and coat the base of the pan. Cook until the eggs are just set, then remove from the heat.

④ Let cool slightly, then stir in the olive oil. Transfer to a serving plate and top with the salmon roe and the reserved spring onion. Serve immediately. Optionally, serve with vegetables and low-carb bread.

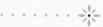 **FUN FACT**

Fish roe contains DHA, the most active type of omega-3. DHA can decrease triglycerides and cardiovascular risk and protect against insulin resistance and type II diabetes. It can also improve learning ability and protect against cognitive decline.

NUTRITION FACTS PER SERVING (SCRAMBLE, NO VEGETABLES OR BREAD):

Total carbs: 6.6 g	Fat: 50.5 g (of which saturated: 15.4 g)	Saturated / MUFA / PUFA (%): 30, 57, 13
Fiber: 0.5 g	Calories: 581 kcal	Omega-6/3 ratio: 0.4 ☺
Net Carbs: 6.1 g	Macronutrient ratio: Calories from carbs (4%), protein (19%), fat (77%)	
Protein: 28.7 g		

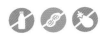
SAUSAGE-AVO-EGG STACK

Commercially available sausage meat is often packed with unwanted preservatives, starches, and even sugar, which means you must steer clear of it—or at least check the label carefully. Luckily, it's easy to make your own! Try our version, which is full of warming spices and fresh herbs, then use it to make this fun-to-eat breakfast stack, which is layered with creamy avocado and choline-rich fried eggs.

HOMEMADE SAUSAGE MEAT

1.2 pounds (500 g) ground outdoor-reared pork (10% fat)

2 cloves garlic, minced

2 tablespoons (14 g/0.5 oz) flax meal

2 tablespoons (6 g/0.2 oz) chopped fresh mint

2 teaspoons (2 g) chopped fresh sage leaves or 1 teaspoon dried sage

1 teaspoon chopped fresh rosemary or ½ teaspoon dried rosemary

½ teaspoon fennel seeds

⅛ teaspoon ground cloves

⅛ teaspoon ground nutmeg

1 tablespoon (15 ml) apple cider vinegar

½ teaspoon salt

½ teaspoon black pepper

AVOCADO-EGG-SAUSAGE STACK

¼ recipe Homemade Sausage Meat (125 g/4.4 oz)

1 teaspoon extra-virgin avocado oil or ghee

½ large or 1 small (100 g/3.5 oz) avocado

¼ small (15 g/0.5 oz) red onion, diced

1 tablespoon (15 ml) fresh lime or lemon juice

1 tablespoon (15 ml) extra-virgin olive oil

Salt and black pepper, to taste

1 large egg

Optional: pinch of chile flakes

① To make the sausage meat: Place all the ingredients in a bowl and mix well. Use one-quarter (125 g/4.4 oz) of the mixture to create a small sausage patty. Store the leftover sausage meat in the fridge for up to 1 day or freeze for up to 3 months.

② To make the stacks: Grease a skillet with the avocado oil over medium heat. Place the patty in the pan and cook undisturbed for 2 to 3 minutes. Flip over and cook for 1 to 2 minutes and set aside.

③ Meanwhile, halve the avocado and scoop into a bowl. Add the onion, lime juice, olive oil, salt, and pepper. Mash using a fork and set aside.

④ Fry the egg in the rendered sausage fat until the white is cooked through and the yolk is still runny.

⑤ To assemble: Top the patty with the prepared guacamole and fried egg. Season with salt and pepper to taste, and a pinch of chile flakes if desired. Eat immediately.

FUN FACT

Two hundred grams of pork contains more than 100 percent of your RDA of selenium, a mineral that supports healthy thyroid function and serves as the core of antioxidant enzymes called selenoproteins.

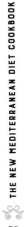

NUTRITION FACTS PER SERVING (1 STACK):

Total carbs: 13.5 g	Fat: 44.1 g (of which saturated: 8 g)	Saturated / MUFA / PUFA (%): 18, 70, 12
Fiber: 8.4 g	Calories: 576 kcal	Omega-6/3 ratio: 3.3
Net Carbs: 5.1 g	Macronutrient ratio: Calories from carbs (4%), protein (26%), fat (70%)	
Protein: 35.8 g		

HERB & CHEESE FRITTERS

These veggie fritters are just as good cold as they are hot, so they're perfect for on-the-go breakfasts and packable lunches. Spread them with mashed avocado, or, if you have a little extra time, a fried egg. They also make an excellent quick snack: serve them with some homemade mayo or aioli (page 199).

3 medium (1.3 pounds/600 g) zucchini

8 ounces (225 g) frozen spinach, thawed and squeezed dry (weight excludes water squeezed out)

4 large eggs

½ teaspoon salt

¼ teaspoon black pepper

3 tablespoons (21 g/0.7 oz) flax meal or coconut flour

¼ cup (20 g/0.7 oz) grated Pecorino Romano

2 cloves garlic, minced

¼ cup (15 g/0.5 oz) chopped fresh herbs, such as parsley, basil, oregano, mint, chives, and/or thyme

¼ cup (60 ml) extra-virgin avocado oil or ghee

① Grate the zucchini and place in a bowl lined with cheesecloth. Set aside for 5 minutes, then twist the cheesecloth around the zucchini and squeeze out as much liquid as you can. You should end up with about 13 ounces (370 g) of drained zucchini.

② In a mixing bowl, combine the zucchini, spinach, eggs, salt, and pepper. Add the flax meal and Pecorino and stir again. Add the garlic and herbs and mix through.

③ Heat a large pan greased with 1 tablespoon (15 ml) of ghee over medium heat. Once hot, use a ¼-cup (60 ml) measuring cup to make the fritters (about 57 g/2 oz each). Place in the hot pan and shape with a spatula. Cook in batches for 3 to 4 minutes per side, until crisp and golden. Grease the pan between each batch until all the ghee has been used.

④ Eat warm or cold, as a breakfast, side, or snack. Store in the fridge for up to 4 days or freeze for up to 3 months.

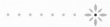 **FUN FACT**

Spinach is a super-low-carb veg, which makes it a great addition to a Mediterranean-keto diet. However, it is high in oxalates, compounds that can bind to minerals in the gut, such as calcium, keeping the body from absorbing them and contributing to the formation of kidney stones. If you're concerned about oxalate content, pre-boiling your spinach can reduce its oxalate content by 60 percent.

NUTRITION FACTS PER SERVING (3 FRITTERS):

Total carbs: 7.9 g	Fat: 18.5 g (of which saturated: 3.5 g)	Saturated / MUFA / PUFA (%): 19, 64, 17
Fiber: 3.8 g	Calories: 231 kcal	Omega-6/3 ratio: 1.7 ☺
Net Carbs: 4.1 g	Macronutrient ratio: Calories from carbs (7%), protein (19%), fat (74%)	
Protein: 10.5 g		

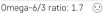

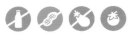

SUNDAY FRITTATA MUFFINS, THREE WAYS

Traditional frittatas require a little fuss: they have to be cooked on the stovetop in a skillet before being baked in the oven. Plus, they often involve potatoes, which certainly aren't low-carb. These brunch-worthy keto egg muffins are so much simpler, and you can add any combination of veggies, herbs, and protein. Just combine the ingredients for the batter in a bowl, pour into a muffin tin, and bake. Here are our three favorite ways to make them!

BASE

6 large eggs

Pinch of salt and black pepper

1 tablespoon (15 ml) extra-virgin avocado oil or ghee

SPINACH PESTO MUFFINS

4 ounces (113 g) frozen spinach, thawed and squeezed dry (weight excludes water squeezed out), chopped

¼ cup (25 g/0.9 oz) sliced Kalamata olives

3 tablespoons (45 ml) Macadamia Basil Pesto (page 198)

¼ cup (37 g/1.3 oz) finely diced red bell pepper

¼ cup (40 g/1.4 oz) finely diced red onion

1 teaspoon dried thyme

3 ounces (85 g) buffalo mozzarella, divided among the number of muffins

CHEESY BROCCOLI MUFFINS

½ medium (200 g/7 oz) broccoli, cut into florets

¾ cup (60 g/2.1 oz) grated Pecorino Romano

¼ cup (40 g/1.4 oz) finely diced red onion

1 tablespoon (3 g/0.1 oz) chopped fresh chives or parsley

1 teaspoon chile flakes

SMOKED SALMON MUFFINS

5 ounces (142 g) frozen spinach, thawed and squeezed dry (weight excludes water squeezed out), chopped

5 ounces (142 g) wild smoked salmon, chopped

2 tablespoons (6 g/0.2 oz) chopped fresh chives or dill

1 teaspoon lemon zest

① Preheat the oven to 360°F (180°C) fan assisted or 400°F (200°C) conventional.

② To make the base: Whisk the eggs with salt and pepper.

③ To make the spinach pesto muffins: Place all of the ingredients apart from the mozzarella in the bowl with the eggs. Stir to combine.

④ To make the cheesy broccoli muffins: Blanch the broccoli in boiling water for 2 to 3 minutes. Using a slotted spoon, immediately transfer to a bowl filled with ice water. Strain and shake off excess water. Chop into 1-inch (2.5 cm) pieces and divide evenly among the individual muffin cups. Mix the eggs with the cheese, onion, chives, and chile flakes.

⑤ To make the smoked salmon muffins: Place all of the ingredients in the bowl with the eggs. Stir to combine.

⑥ To make the muffins: Grease a standard-size muffin tray with the avocado oil and divide the egg mixture evenly among 10 muffin cups. If you're making the Spinach Pesto Muffins, add the mozzarella. Place in the oven and bake for about 20 minutes or until fully set and lightly browned on top.

NUTRITION FACTS PER SERVING (1 SPINACH PESTO/CHEESY BROCCOLI/SMOKED SALMON EGG MUFFIN):

Total carbs: 1.8/2.3/0.9 g	Fat: 9.3/6/5.7 g (of which saturated: 2.5/2.1/1.5 g)	Saturated / MUFA / PUFA (%): 27, 67, 6 / 35, 56, 9 / 20, 67, 13
Fiber: 0.6/0.7/0.5 g	Calories: 117/89/85 kcal	Omega-6/3 ratio: 2.2 / 2.2 / 0.8 ☺
Net Carbs: 1.2/1.6/0.4 g	Macronutrient ratio: Calories from carbs (4/8/2%), protein (23/30/36%), fat (73/62/62%)	
Protein: 6.5/6.6/7.4 g		

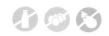

CRUNCHY VANILLA PROTEIN BARS

Ideal for busy mornings, post-workout refueling, and snacking on the go, these clean protein bars aren't like anything you can buy on supermarket shelves. Their macros are perfectly proportioned, with 76% fat, 20% protein, and only 4% carbs. Munch two as a meal replacement when you're in a rush.

TOPPING

½ cup (30 g/1.1 oz) flaked coconut

2 tablespoons (28 g/1 oz) raw cacao nibs

BARS

1½ cups (150 g/3.5 oz) almond flour

1 cup (100 g/3.5 oz) collagen powder

2 tablespoons (16 g/0.6 oz) ground or whole chia seeds

1 teaspoon vanilla powder or 1 tablespoon (15 ml) unsweetened vanilla extract

¼ cup (60 ml) virgin coconut oil

½ cup (120 ml) coconut milk

1½ teaspoons fresh lemon zest

⅓ cup (45 g/1.6 oz) macadamia nuts, halved

Optional: low-carb sweetener, to taste

① Preheat the oven to 350°F (175°C) fan assisted or 380°F (195°C) conventional.

② To make the topping: Place the coconut flakes on a baking tray and bake for 2 to 3 minutes, until lightly golden. Set aside to cool.

③ To make the bars: In a bowl, combine all of the ingredients for the bars. Line a small baking tray with parchment paper or use a silicone baking tray. A square 8 × 8–inch (20 × 20 cm) or a rectangular tray of similar size will work best.

④ Press the dough into the pan and sprinkle with the cacao nibs, pressing them into the bars with your fingers. Add the toasted coconut and lightly press the flakes into the dough. Refrigerate until set, for about 1 hour. Slice to serve. Store in the refrigerator for up to 1 week.

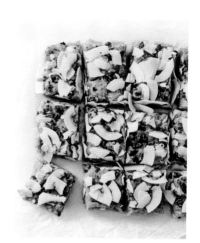

NUTRITION FACTS PER SERVING (1 BAR):

Total carbs: 7.6 g

Fiber: 4.2 g

Net Carbs: 3.4 g

Protein: 16.6 g

Fat: 28.7 g (of which saturated: 13.1 g)

Calories: 338 kcal

Macronutrient ratio: Calories from carbs (4%), protein (20%), fat (76%)

SAT / MUFA / PUFA (%): 47, 37, 16

Omega-6/3 ratio: 1.6 ☺

BREAKFASTS

ON-THE-GO SAVORY GRANOLA BARS, TWO WAYS

Brace yourself for a revelation: Granola bars don't have to be sweet. (Mind = blown.) Think of our savory granola bars as your favorite roasted nuts packed in a travel-friendly snack. We love these garlic-and-herb and curried versions, but you can use any nuts, seeds, herbs, and spices you have on hand. Stash a few in a sealed container in your car or at your desk at work.

BASIC BARS

2 cups (200 g/7 oz) pecans

⅓ cup (83 g/3 oz) tahini

¼ cup (36 g/1.3 oz) sesame seeds

1 large egg

1 teaspoon salt

1 teaspoon black pepper

GARLIC & HERB

1 teaspoon chile flakes

1 teaspoon dried Italian herbs

½ teaspoon garlic powder

1 ounce (28 g) chopped sun-dried tomatoes

1 teaspoon onion powder

2 tablespoons (24 g/0.8 oz) nutritional yeast

1 tablespoon (15 ml) water

CURRIED

1 teaspoon ground turmeric

2 teaspoons (5 g) ground cumin

½ teaspoon ground coriander

1 clove garlic, minced

1 teaspoon onion powder

① Preheat the oven to 285°F (140°C) fan assisted or 320°F (160°C) conventional.

② Roughly chop the pecans or place in a food processor and pulse until chopped but still chunky. Place the pecans in a bowl add the remaining ingredients for your variation of choice.

③ Use your fingers to press the mixture into a medium baking dish (about 8 × 8 inch [20 × 20 cm]); use a silicone baking dish or a regular baking dish lined with parchment paper. Bake for about 25 minutes or until crispy. Remove from the pan and allow to cool slightly. Slice into 8 bars with a greased sharp knife. Store in a sealed container for up to 3 days or freeze for up to 3 months.

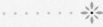 **FUN FACT**

Granola bars are great for fueling exercise. Aerobic exercise can increase the expression of the anti-aging protein SIRT3 in your brain! SIRT3 activates antioxidant (SOD2) and fat-burning enzymes, and protects against Alzheimer's disease in animal models.

NUTRITION FACTS PER SERVING (1 GARLIC & HERB/CURRIED GRANOLA BAR):

Total carbs: 9.6/7.8 g	Fat: 27/26.4 g (of which saturated: 2.9/2.8 g)	Saturated / MUFA / PUFA (%): 11, 52, 37 / 11, 52, 37
Fiber: 5.2/4.2 g	Calories: 290/273 kcal	Omega-6: 9.5 g. Remember, sesame and tahini break the omega-6 rule because of sesame's lignan antioxidants!
Net Carbs: 4.4/3.6 g	Macronutrient ratio: Calories from carbs (6/5%), protein (10/8%), fat (84/87%)	
Protein: 7.5/5.8 g		

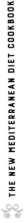

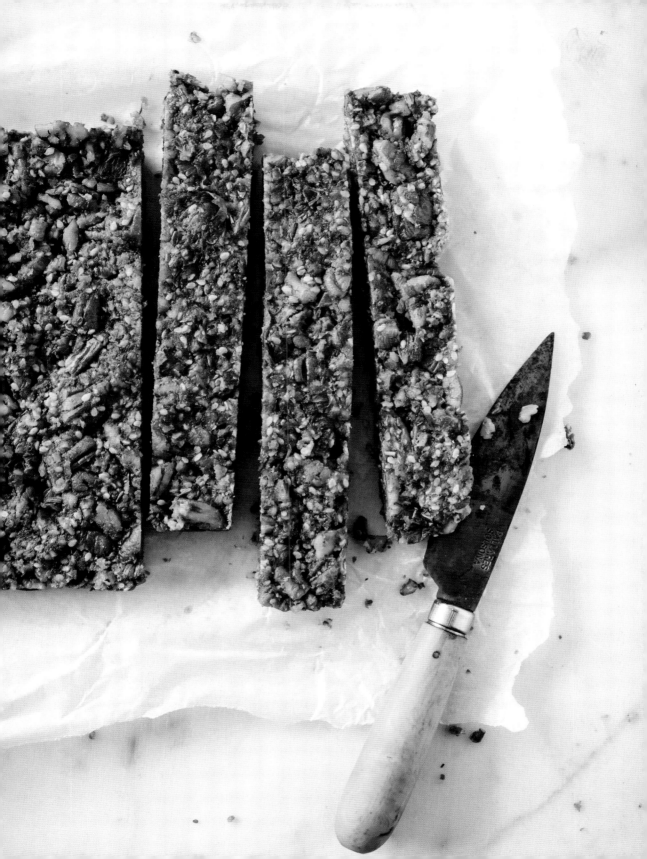

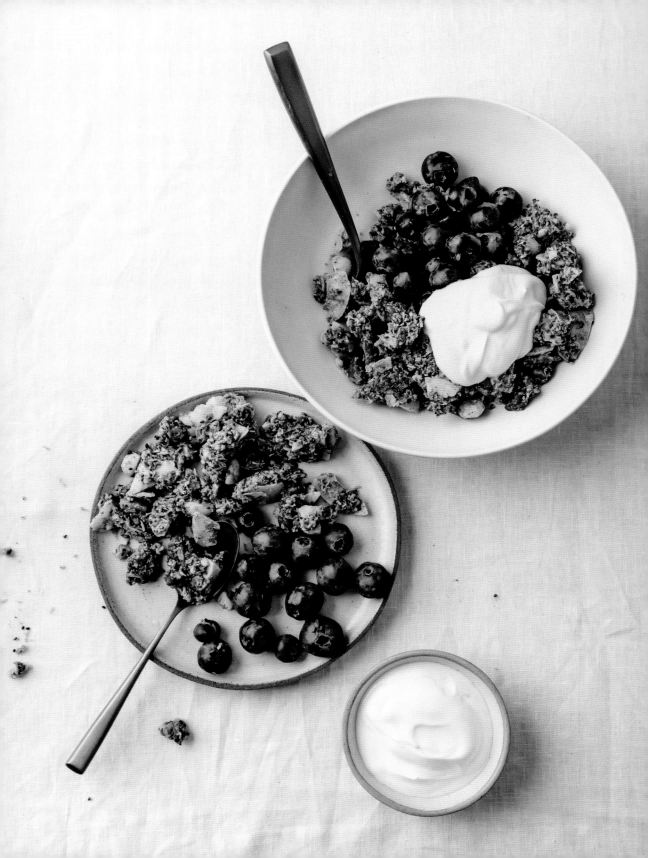

SERVINGS:
10 (5 cups)

HANDS-ON TIME:
10 minutes

OVERALL TIME:
1 hour 20 minutes

SPICED ANTIOXIDANT GRANOLA CLUSTERS

This crunchy granola is packed with so many antioxidants it's nuts! (Sorry, we couldn't resist.) We use coconut, pecans, and blanched almonds, but feel free to substitute your favorites. Macadamia is a great option, due to its high MUFA content and anti-inflammatory qualities. No need to add any sweeteners here, either: warming spices like cinnamon, ginger, and anise add a subtle sweetness of their own.

1 cup (75 g/2.7 oz) unsweetened fine coconut flakes

1 cup (60 g/2.1 oz) unsweetened large coconut flakes

¼ cup packed (38 g/1.3 oz) flax meal

¼ cup (38 g/1.3 oz) chia seeds

½ cup (50 g/1.8 oz) pecans, chopped

1 cup (145 g/5.1 oz) blanched almonds, roughly chopped, or flaked almonds

2 teaspoons (5 g) cinnamon

1 teaspoon ground anise seed

½ teaspoon ground nutmeg

½ teaspoon ground cloves

1 tablespoon (6 g/0.2 oz) fresh lemon zest

¼ teaspoon black pepper

¼ teaspoon salt

⅓ cup (83 g/3 oz) light tahini

¼ cup (60 ml) virgin coconut oil

2 large egg whites

Optional: unsweetened almond milk, coconut cream, coconut yogurt, or full-fat goat's yogurt, to serve

① Preheat the oven to 265°F (130°C) conventional or 230°F (110°C) fan assisted convection. Line a baking tray with parchment paper.

② Place all of the dry ingredients, including the lemon zest, in a large bowl. Stir to combine. In a small bowl, mix the tahini with the coconut oil, then add to the dry ingredients. Add the egg whites and mix to combine.

③ Spoon onto the lined baking tray and crumble all over. Bake for 1 hour and 10 minutes to 1 hour and 20 minutes, until golden. Remove from the oven and let cool completely; it will crisp up as it cools. Serve on its own or with almond milk, coconut cream or coconut yogurt, or full-fat goat's yogurt. Store in a jar at room temperature for up to 2 weeks or freeze for up to 3 months.

NUTRITION FACTS PER SERVING (½ CUP/50 G/1.8 OZ):

Total carbs: 11.8 g
Fiber: 7.7 g
Net Carbs: 4.1 g
Protein: 9.1 g

Fat: 28.8 g (of which saturated: 10.6 g)
Calories: 329 kcal
Macronutrient ratio: Calories from carbs (5%), protein (12%), fat (83%)

SAT / MUFA / PUFA (%): 37, 33, 30
Omega-6: 5.1 g. Remember, sesame-based tahini breaks the omega-6 rule because of its lignan antioxidants!

BREAKFASTS

59

CREAMY CINNAMON PORRIDGE

If you've been missing high-carb comfort foods like hot cereals, you'll want to treat yourself to a batch of this rich, satisfying breakfast porridge. Bursting with nuts, seeds, and high-quality fats, it gets the sweet treatment from cinnamon, crunchy coconut flakes, and cacao nibs. It sounds almost too indulgent to be good for you, but it was designed especially by Martina—who has a history of thyroid disorders herself—to help support both thyroid function and a healthy metabolism.

¼ cup (60 ml) coconut milk

¾ cup (180 ml) unsweetened almond milk or water

¼ cup (63 g/2.2 oz) almond butter or hazelnut butter

1 tablespoon (15 ml) virgin coconut oil

2 tablespoons (16 g/0.6 oz) chia seeds

1 tablespoon (7 g/0.3 oz) flax meal

1 teaspoon cinnamon

¼ cup (35 g/1.2 oz) macadamia nuts

¼ cup (28 g/1 oz) hazelnuts

4 Brazil nuts (14 g/0.5 oz)

Optional: low-carb sweetener, to taste

¼ cup (15 g/0.5 oz) unsweetened large coconut flakes

1 tablespoon (14 g/0.5 oz) cacao nibs

① In a small saucepan, mix the coconut milk and almond milk and heat over medium heat. Once hot (not boiling), take off the heat. Add the almond butter and coconut oil. Stir until well combined. If needed, use an immersion blender and process until smooth.

② Add the chia seeds, flax meal, and cinnamon, and leave to rest for 5 to 10 minutes. Roughly chop the macadamias, hazelnuts, and Brazil nuts and stir in. Add sweetener, if using, and stir. Transfer to serving bowls. In a small skillet, dry-roast the coconut flakes over medium-high heat for 1 to 2 minutes, until lightly toasted and fragrant. Top the porridge with the toasted coconut flakes and cacao nibs (or you can use chopped 100% chocolate). Serve immediately or store in the fridge for up to 3 days.

FUN FACT

Selenium, zinc, and magnesium are three micronutrients essential to thyroid health. Brazil nuts are the world's best source of selenium: just a single nut contains your entire RDA! Seeds and nuts are generally rich in zinc, while flax meal, coconut milk, and cacao nibs are all great sources of magnesium. Try the Salmon Fish Cakes with Fennel "Noodles" and Brazil Nut Pesto on page 118, too: it's also been designed to promote thyroid function.

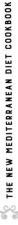

NUTRITION FACTS PER SERVING (1 BOWL):

Total carbs: 21 g	Fat: 69.7 g (of which saturated: 23.2 g)	Saturated / MUFA / PUFA (%): 33, 51, 16
Fiber: 12.7 g	Calories: 727 kcal	Omega-6/3 ratio: 1.2 ☺
Net Carbs: 8.3 g	Macronutrient ratio: Calories from carbs (5%), protein (9%), fat (86%)	
Protein: 15.7 g		

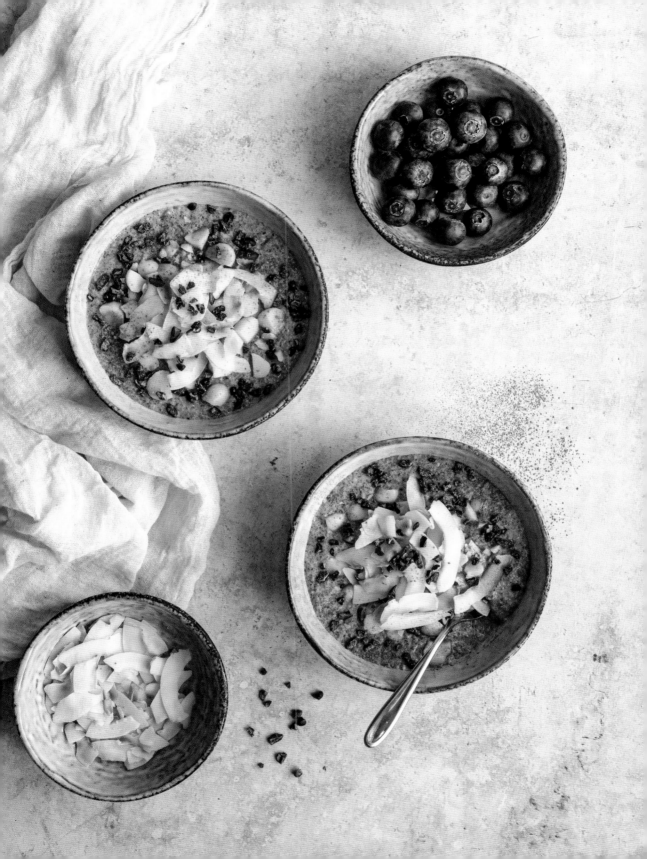

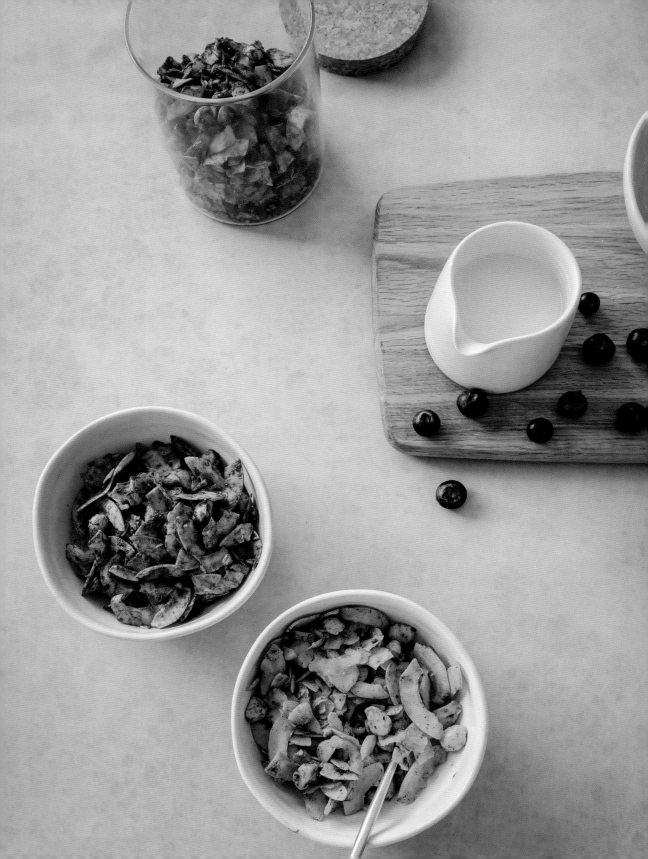

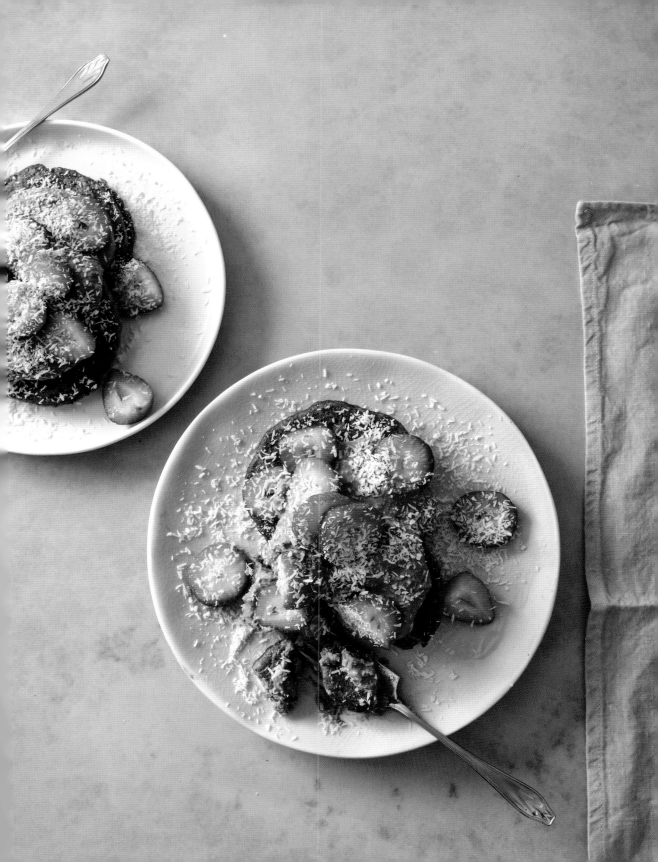

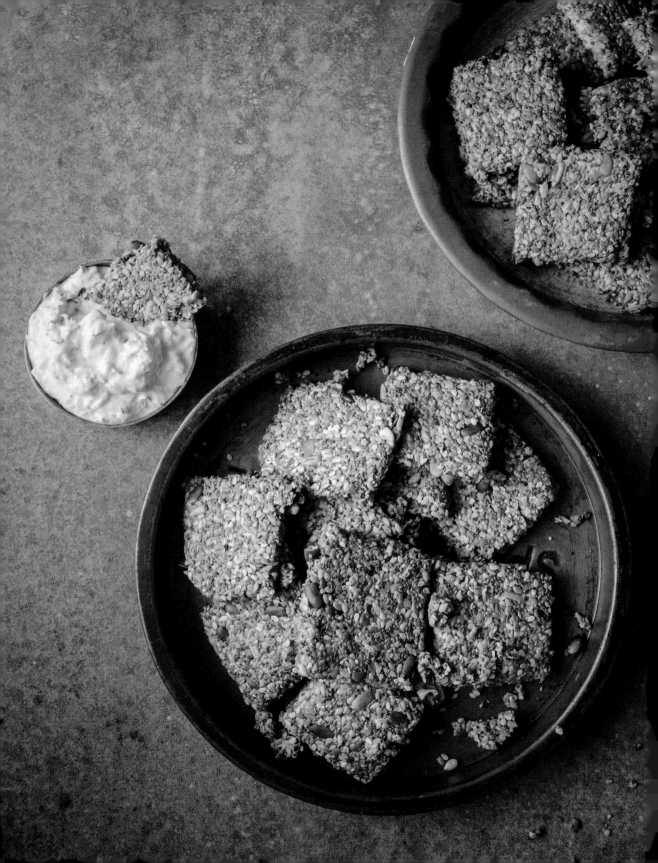

CHAPTER 3

SNACKS

SUPERSEED CRACKERS, TWO WAYS

To "supersede" means "to take the place of." You'll never crave store-bought crackers again. Keep them simple with just salt and pepper—or try nutritional yeast to add a cheesy umami twist. Toss in some turmeric, along with other Mediterranean spices, to add a golden color and extra anti-inflammatory power.

BASIC CRACKERS

⅓ cup (47 g/1.6 oz) sunflower seeds

⅓ cup (48 g/1.7 oz) sesame seeds

⅓ cup (56 g/2 oz) flaxseeds

¼ cup (38 g/1.3 oz) chia seeds

⅓ cup (43 g/1.5 oz) pumpkin seeds

2 tablespoons (18 g/0.6 oz) poppy seeds

1 teaspoon coarse black pepper

1 teaspoon salt

1 cup (240 ml) water

CHEESY CRACKERS

3 tablespoons (36 g/1.3 oz) nutritional yeast

1 teaspoon garlic powder

2 teaspoons (3 g) dried Italian herbs

4–6 pieces (28 g/1 oz) sun-dried tomatoes, finely chopped

GOLDEN CRACKERS

1 teaspoon ground turmeric

1 teaspoon ground cumin

1 teaspoon onion powder

½ teaspoon chile flakes or ¼ teaspoon chile powder

¼ teaspoon ground coriander

① Preheat the oven to 285°F (140°C) fan assisted or 320°F (160°C) conventional.

② To make the basic crackers: Place all the ingredients for the basic crackers, apart from the water, in a bowl. Combine well. Place about ½ cup (75 g) of the mixture into a food processor and process until finely ground, scraping down the sides of the food processor as needed. Return the ground seed mixture to the bowl.

③ Add the remaining ingredients for your recipe of choice and stir until well combined. Finally, add the water. Mix with a spoon until well combined, then let the mixture sit for 5 to 10 minutes.

④ Place a silicone mat or a piece of heavy-duty parchment paper in a 10 × 14–inch (25 × 35 cm) baking tray. Transfer the dough to the tray and spread with a rubber spatula, shaping it into the rectangular shape of the silicone mat, until it is about ⅛ inch (3 mm) thick. Use a pizza cutter to cut it into 24 crackers (6 rows by 4 columns).

⑤ Bake for 50 to 60 minutes, until crispy and golden brown. When done, remove from the oven, and cut through the precut crackers. Let them cool down and crisp up on a cooling rack for 20 to 30 minutes before serving. Store for up to 2 weeks at room temperature in a sealed container.

NUTRITION FACTS PER CRACKER (CHEESY/GOLDEN):

Total carbs: 3.7/2.9 g	Fat: 4.9/4.7 g (of which saturated: 0.6/0.6 g)	Saturated / MUFA / PUFA (%): 13, 26, 61 / 13, 26, 61
Fiber: 2.4/2 g	Calories: 66/59 kcal	Omega-6/3 ratio: 1.4 / 1.4 ☺
Net Carbs: 1.3/0.9 g	Macronutrient ratio: Calories from carbs (9/7%), protein (20/16%), fat (71/77%)	
Protein: 3/2.2 g		

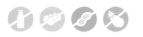

TARAMASALATA

Taramasalata is a traditional Mediterranean dip served in almost every Greek *taverna*. Traditional taramasalata blends bread or potatoes with omega-3-rich smoked cod roe (*tarama*), lemon juice, vinegar, and olive oil. Our ketogenic version trades the bread's carbs for cauliflower's vitamin C and choline, and if you ask us, it's even more delicious than the original!

1 small (400 g/14.1 oz) cauliflower, cut into florets

8.8 ounces (250 g) smoked cod roe

¼ cup (60 ml) fresh lemon juice, divided

2 tablespoons (30 ml) apple cider vinegar, divided

1 cup (240 ml) plus 2 tablespoons (30 ml) extra-virgin olive oil, divided

½ teaspoon black pepper

Optional: Superseed Crackers (page 70), celery sticks, sliced cucumber, bell peppers, and Kalamata olives, to serve

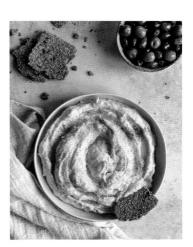

① Place the cauliflower florets in a steamer pot filled with 1 cup (240 ml) water and cover with a lid. Bring to a boil and cook over medium-high heat until soft, for 12 to 15 minutes. Remove the lid to let the steam escape and let the cauliflower cool to room temperature.

② Cut the smoked cod roe into smaller pieces. (Sometimes it comes wrapped in a thin foil that you will need to peel off.) Place in a food processor with about 2 tablespoons (30 ml) of the lemon juice, 1 tablespoon (15 ml) of the apple cider vinegar, and ¼ cup (60 ml) of the extra-virgin olive oil. Process until combined, then add the remaining 2 tablespoons (30 ml) lemon juice and 1 tablespoon (15 ml) vinegar. Process again until combined.

③ Add the cooked and cooled cauliflower florets and black pepper. Start blending, slowly drizzling in ¾ cup (180 ml) olive oil as you do so. The taramasalata is ready when there are no visible pieces left and the mixture is smooth and creamy.

④ Transfer to a bowl, drizzle with the remaining 2 tablespoons (30 ml) olive oil, and serve. To store, place in a sealed container and refrigerate for up to 1 week.

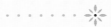 **FUN FACT**

Fish eggs, or roe, are the world's richest source of lyso-DHA, the best form of the best type of omega-3 for the brain. Lyso-DHA in particular can help ward off Alzheimer's disease because it gets privileged access to the brain via the MSFD2A transporter!

NUTRITION FACTS PER SERVING (ABOUT ½ CUP/120 G/4.2 OZ):

Total carbs: 3.2 g	Fat: 30.6 g (of which saturated: 4.3 g)	Saturated / MUFA / PUFA (%): 14, 74, 12
Fiber: 1.1 g	Calories: 323 kcal	Omega-6/3 ratio: 4.0. The absolute omega-6/3 ratio matters less on this dish, which is about omega-3 quality. It's a rare source of lyso-DHA!
Net Carbs: 2.1 g	Macronutrient ratio: Calories from carbs (3%), protein (13%), fat (84%)	
Protein: 10.6 g		

FENNEL TZATZIKI

(CONTRIBUTOR: NINA TEICHOLZ)

Here's another quintessential Greek dip! This one was contributed by Nina Teicholz, a Stanford- and Oxford-trained journalist who has become one of the world's most prominent advocates of the evidence-based perspective that saturated fat does not cause heart disease. That means there's no reason not to indulge in this classic creamy yogurt dip, made with fresh cucumber, herbs, and lemon, plus a liquorishy fennel twist to boost heart health. Serve it alongside raw low-carb veggies or Superseed Crackers (page 70) or try it with our souvlaki (page 150).

1 medium (150 g/5.3 oz) cucumber

½ small (85 g/3 oz) fennel bulb

2 cups (500 g/1.1 lb) full-fat 100% sheep's or goat's milk yogurt

5 tablespoons (75 ml) extra-virgin olive oil, divided

2 tablespoons (30 ml) fresh lemon juice

1 teaspoon finely grated fresh lemon zest

1 clove garlic, crushed

2 tablespoons (3 g) chopped fresh dill

Salt and black pepper, to taste

① Grate the cucumber and place it in a bowl. Drain any excess juices. Finely slice the fennel, or place in a food processor and use a slicing blade to process until finely sliced. Add it to the bowl with the cucumber. Add the yogurt, 3 tablespoons (45 ml) of the olive oil, lemon juice, lemon zest, garlic, dill, salt, and pepper. Stir to combine and drizzle with the remaining 2 tablespoons (30 ml) olive oil. Store in the fridge in a sealed jar for up to 5 days.

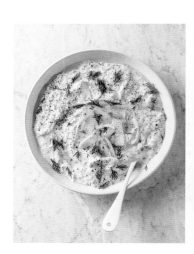

☀ FUN FACT ☀

The *Journal of the American College of Cardiology* states there are "no beneficial effects of reducing saturated fat intake on cardiovascular disease," but rather that saturated fat intake may be protective against stroke.

NUTRITION FACTS PER SERVING (ABOUT ⅔ CUP/140 G/5 OZ):

Total carbs: 6.4 g	Fat: 19.7 g (of which saturated: 7 g)	Saturated / MUFA / PUFA (%): 36, 56, 8
Fiber: 0.7 g	Calories: 223 kcal	Omega-6: 1.5 g
Net Carbs: 5.7 g	Macronutrient ratio: Calories from carbs (10%), protein (11%), fat (79%)	
Protein: 6.4 g		

SAVORY MACKEREL & GOAT'S CHEESE "PARADOX" BALLS

The French consume 58 pounds (26.3 kg) of cheese per person per year, yet their rate of heart disease is surprisingly low. This so-called "French Paradox" may be due, in part, to the heart-healthy qualities of certain cheeses, such as goat's cheese. Here, we add omega-3-rich mackerel to soft goat's cheese for the creamiest ever fish pâté; then we roll it in manganese-rich pecans for a fast, high-fat, low-fuss snack.

2 smoked or cooked mackerel fillets (200 g/7 oz), boneless, skin removed

4.4 ounces (125 g) soft goat's cheese

1 tablespoon (15 ml) fresh lemon juice

1 teaspoon Dijon or yellow mustard

1 small (60 g/2.1 oz) red onion, finely diced

2 tablespoons (6 g/0.2 oz) chopped fresh chives or herbs of choice

¾ cup (85 g/3 oz) pecans, crushed

10 leaves (85 g/3 oz) baby gem lettuce

① In a food processor, combine the mackerel, goat's cheese, lemon juice, and mustard. Pulse until smooth. Transfer to a bowl, add the onion and herbs, and mix with a spoon. Refrigerate for 20 to 30 minutes, or until set.

② Using a large spoon or an ice cream scoop, divide the mixture into 10 balls, about 40 g/1.4 ounces each. Roll each ball in the crushed pecans. Place each ball on a small lettuce leaf and serve. Keep the fat bombs refrigerated in a sealed container for up to 5 days.

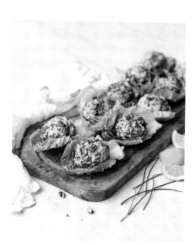

 FUN FACT

It's much healthier to indulge and then fast than it is to graze. Not only does it help cut body fat, but fasting can also promote intermittent metabolic switching in your brain, making you more resistant to cognitive decline. Eating each day within a six- or eight-hour window is a smart move for most people, and it makes the meals you do have more indulgent, too!

NUTRITION FACTS PER SERVING (1 FAT BOMB):

Total carbs: 1.9 g	Fat: 13.1 g (of which saturated: 3.6 g)	Saturated / MUFA / PUFA (%): 27, 48, 25
Fiber: 1 g	Calories: 151 kcal	Omega-6/3 ratio: 2.4
Net Carbs: 0.9 g	Macronutrient ratio: Calories from carbs (2%), protein (20%), fat (78%)	
Protein: 7.5 g		

4:1 HUMMUS

(CONTRIBUTOR: DR. CHRIS PALMER)

The 4 parts fat to 1 part protein plus carbs diet is an extra-fatty ketogenic diet used to treat neurological disorders. This "hummus" was contributed by Dr. Chris Palmer, a Harvard psychiatrist and the world's leading expert on using ketogenic diets for mental health. Dr. Palmer says, "The 4:1 diet can be difficult to follow, but delicious recipes like this one make it easier. Keep a batch of this spread on hand in your fridge: it's delicious on anything. Its versatility is what makes it such a powerful medical treatment!"

TO SOAK

1 cup (134 g/4.7 oz) macadamia nuts

TO ROAST

2 medium (400 g/14.1 oz) zucchini

2 tablespoons (30 ml) extra-virgin avocado oil

TO BLEND

¼ cup (64 g/2.2 oz) tahini

2 cloves garlic, minced

¼ cup (60 ml) fresh lemon juice

2 tablespoons (30 ml) extra-virgin olive oil

1 teaspoon ground cumin

Fresh herbs, such as parsley or cilantro

Salt and black pepper, to taste

TOPPING

2 tablespoons (30 ml) extra-virgin olive oil

Pinch of paprika and/or ground cumin

1 tablespoon (9 g/0.3 oz) white and/ or black sesame seeds

① To soak: Place the macadamias in a bowl and add enough filtered water to cover them. Soak for about 2 hours, and then drain and discard the water.

② To roast: Meanwhile, preheat the oven to 320°F (160°C) fan assisted or 355°F (180°C) conventional. Cut off the ends of the zucchini and cut in half lengthwise.

③ Arrange on a baking tray, cut-side up, and brush with the of avocado oil. Bake for 30 minutes or until browned on top.

④ To blend: Add all the ingredients, apart from the topping ingredients, to a food processor. Blend until smooth. Season with salt and pepper to taste.

⑤ Transfer to a bowl and add the topping: drizzle with the olive oil and sprinkle with paprika and sesame seeds. Store in a sealed container in the fridge for up to 5 days or freeze for up to 3 months. To defrost, place in the fridge overnight.

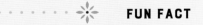 **FUN FACT**

Dr. Palmer treated an eighty-two-year-old woman with a fifty-three-year history of schizophrenia who suffered from symptoms such as paranoia and hallucinations. In 2008 she began a ketogenic diet. Within two weeks, her symptoms had improved, and she was eventually able to stop taking all her psychiatric medications. She remains on the diet, and has been symptom-free for fourteen years.

NUTRITION FACTS PER SERVING (ABOUT ¼ CUP/57 G/2 OZ):

Total carbs: 4.5 g	Fat: 18.7 g (of which saturated: 2.7 g)	Saturated / MUFA / PUFA (%): 14, 73, 13
Fiber: 2 g	Calories: 185 kcal	Omega-6: 2.25 g. Remember, sesame/ tahini breaks the omega-6 rule because of its lignan antioxidants!
Net Carbs: 2.5 g	Macronutrient ratio: Calories from carbs (5%), protein (5%), fat (90%)	
Protein: 2.4 g		

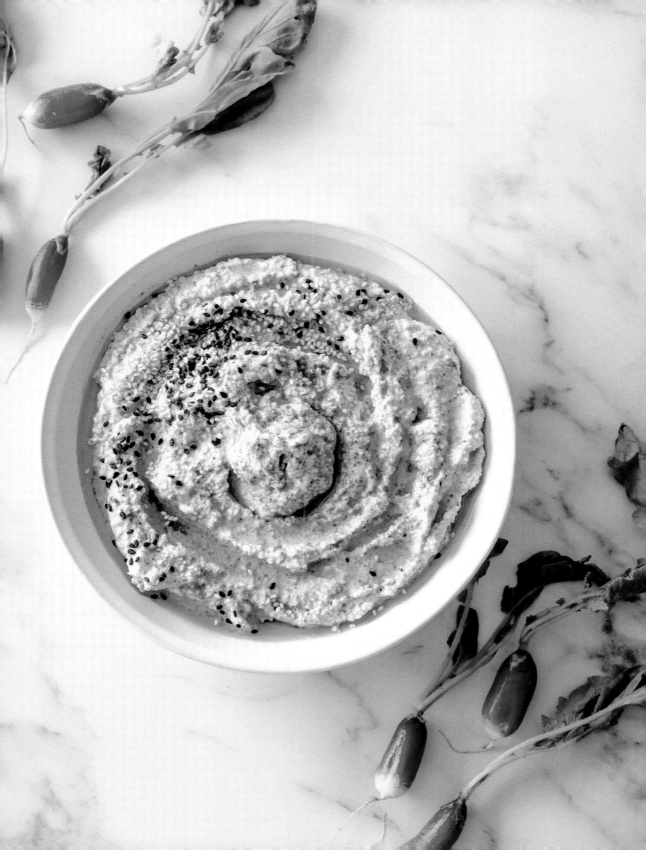

A+ CHICKEN LIVER PÂTÉ

This classic vitamin A-rich chicken liver pâté is flavored with fresh herbs, garlic, onion, and mustard, and it definitely scores an A+ when it comes to nutrition. As one of the runners-up in our list of high-fat superfoods for your Mediterranean-keto diet, it's also high in riboflavin, folate, vitamin B_{12}, and selenium. It also happens to be the perfect party food: a great partner for Superseed Crackers (page 70) or Quick Low-Carb Bread (page 38).

2 tablespoons (30 ml) ghee, plus more for storage

1 small (60 g/2.1 oz) red onion, diced

3 cloves garlic, minced

1.1 pounds (500 g) raw chicken livers or other liver

2 tablespoons (5 g/0.2 oz) fresh thyme leaves, plus more for topping

1 tablespoon (3 g/0.1 oz) chopped fresh sage leaves, plus more for topping

¼ cup (60 ml) extra-virgin olive oil

1 tablespoon (15 ml) Dijon or yellow mustard

Salt and black pepper, to taste

Optional: Superseed Crackers (page 70) or Focaccia (page 179), to serve; cooked, crumbled crispy bacon pieces, for topping

① Heat a skillet greased with 2 tablespoons (30 ml) of ghee over medium heat. Sauté the onion for about 3 minutes, until fragrant, then add the garlic.

② Use a knife to cut out the sinews from the liver, then chop the liver into about 1-inch (2.5 cm) pieces. Add to the pan and cook for 5 to 7 minutes, stirring frequently. They should be opaque and just cooked. (Do not over-cook or the livers will become tough and dry.)

③ Stir in the herbs and cook for 2 to 3 minutes. Remove the skillet from the heat and let it rest for about 10 minutes. Place the liver mixture and all the other ingredients, apart from the remaining ghee, in a blender. Process until smooth and creamy.

④ Serve immediately with crackers or focaccia, or on its own. Optionally, top with crispy bacon pieces.

⑤ To store, place in a sealed container and top with about 2 tablespoons (30 ml) melted ghee, or enough to completely cover the pâté; this will make it last for longer. Add a few sprigs of thyme and a few sage leaves. Place in the fridge and store for up to 1 week. Remove from the fridge at least 30 minutes before serving.

NUTRITION FACTS PER SERVING (¼ CUP/57 G/2 OZ):

Total carbs: 1.4 g	Fat: 8.2 g (of which saturated: 3 g)	Saturated / MUFA / PUFA (%): 37, 54, 9
Fiber: 0.2 g	Calories: 118 kcal	Omega-6: 0.9 g
Net Carbs: 1.2 g	Macronutrient ratio: Calories from carbs (4%), protein (31%), fat (65%)	
Protein: 8.7 g		

OAT'S CHEESE & HAZELNUT DIP

his lemony, lightly herbed French-style dip is perfect for just about any get-together: ames nights, cocktail parties, baby showers, you name it. It takes just a few minutes o prepare (even less if you have a food processor). Serve it with Superseed Crackers page 70), sliced vegetable sticks, or, as we suggest here, crisp, bitter chicory or ndive leaves.

heads (250 g/8.8 oz) yellow
hicory or endive

nough ice water to cover the leaves

inch of salt

IP

2 ounces (340 g) soft goat's cheese

tablespoons (45 ml) extra-virgin
live oil

tablespoon (15 ml) fresh
emon juice

teaspoon lemon zest (about
 lemon)

clove garlic, minced

reshly ground black pepper,
 taste

alt, if needed, to taste

OPPING

tablespoons (6 g/0.2 oz) chopped
esh chives

 cup (28 g/1 oz) crushed hazelnuts,
ecans, or walnuts

tablespoon (15 ml) extra-virgin
live oil

hile flakes or black pepper, to taste

① Cut off the bottom of the chicory and trim the leaves to get rid of any that are limp or brown. Place the leaves in salted ice water for 10 minutes. This will help the chicory leaves to become crisp. Drain and leave in the strainer.

② To make the dip: Place the dip ingredients in a bowl and use a fork or spatula to mix until smooth and creamy.

③ Stir in the chives. Transfer to a serving bowl and top with the crushed hazelnuts, olive oil, and chile flakes. Serve with the crisp chicory leaves. Store in a sealed jar in the fridge for up to 5 days.

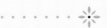 **FUN FACT**

Some fermented and aged cheeses, such as blue cheeses, contain the immune system molecule histamine that's released during an allergic reaction. This is fine for most people, but some people are histamine intolerant. And the enzyme that breaks down histamine, DAO, fluctuates with the menstrual cycle. It's lowest during and one week after menses. Soft goat's cheese is a low-histamine cheese!

NUTRITION FACTS PER SERVING (ABOUT ¼ CUP/57 G/2 OZ):

otal carbs: 2.1 g
iber: 1.5 g
let Carbs: 0.6 g
rotein: 8.9 g

Fat: 18 g (of which saturated: 7.3 g)
Calories: 202 kcal
Macronutrient ratio: Calories from carbs (1%), protein (18%), fat (81%)

Saturated / MUFA / PUFA (%): 46, 48, 7
Omega-6: 1.2 g

UPGRADED BABA GHANOUSH

Baba ghanoush, a traditional Middle Eastern dip, is naturally low in carbs, because the basic recipe is nothing more than charred eggplant, tahini, garlic, olive oil, and lemon juice. But we've made it even healthier! This version boasts macadamias, lots of extra-virgin olive oil, and a whopping tablespoonful of turmeric, that antioxidant powerhouse.

½ cup (67 g/2.4 oz) macadamias

Enough filtered water to cover the nuts

3 medium eggplants (750 g/ 1.65 lb), to yield about 600 g/ 1.3 lb edible cooked parts

⅓ cup (83 g/3 oz) tahini

¼ cup (60 ml) fresh lemon juice

2 cloves garlic, roughly chopped

1 teaspoon ground cumin

1 tablespoon (9 g/0.3 oz) ground turmeric

½ teaspoon black pepper

¼ teaspoon chili powder

3 tablespoons (12 g/0.4 oz) chopped fresh parsley, plus more for topping

¼ cup (60 ml) plus 1 tablespoon (15 ml) extra-virgin olive oil, divided

Salt, to taste

Pinch of paprika or chile flakes, for topping

① Place the macadamias in a bowl and add enough water to cover them. Soak for about 2 hours, and then drain and discard the water.

② Place the eggplants on a baking tray lined with parchment paper. Using a fork, prick the skin of each eggplant several times. Place under a broiler for 5 to 8 minutes, until the skin is lightly charred. Turn the tray halfway through.

③ Turn the broiler off and pre-heat the oven to 430°F (220°C) fan assisted or 465°F (240°C) conventional. Bake for 30 to 40 minutes. The eggplants will be wrinkly and very soft inside when they are done. Remove from the oven and set aside until they are cool enough to handle.

④ Slit the eggplants and scoop the flesh out. Discard the skins, stems, and excess juices left in the tray. Place the cooked eggplant flesh in a food processor. Add the soaked macadamias, tahini, lemon juice, garlic, cumin, turmeric, pepper, chili powder, parsley, and ¼ cup (60 ml) of the olive oil. Blend until smooth and creamy. Season with salt to taste.

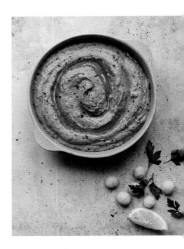

⑤ Transfer to a bowl or a storage container, drizzle with the remaining 1 tablespoon (15 ml) olive oil, and sprinkle with ground paprika and more parsley. To store, seal and refrigerate for up to 5 days.

NUTRITION FACTS PER SERVING (ABOUT ⅓ CUP/85 G/3 OZ):

Total carbs: 8.6 g	Fat: 16.6 g (of which saturated: 2.4 g)	Saturated / MUFA / PUFA (%): 14, 76, 10
Fiber: 4 g	Calories: 183 kcal	Omega-6: 2.75 g. Remember, tahini breaks the omega-6 rule because of its lignan antioxidants!
Net Carbs: 4.6 g	Macronutrient ratio: Calories from carbs (10%), protein (7%), fat (83%)	
Protein: 2.9 g		

ULTIMATE NUT BUTTER

(CONTRIBUTOR: DR. BRIANNA STUBBS)

Gently flavored with cinnamon and vanilla and a diverse source of healthy fats, this recipe for luscious nut butter was contributed by real-life superwoman Dr. Brianna Stubbs, a world rowing champion who became the youngest person ever to row across the English Channel when she was just twelve years old. Today, she holds a Ph.D. from Oxford University and is an acclaimed anti-aging researcher. Brianna, who knows how to fuel her body and brain for optimal performance, eats this Ultimate Nut Butter almost every day.

1½ cups (200 g/7 oz) macadamia nuts

1 cup (100 g/3.5 oz) pecans

½ cup (125 g/4.4 oz) coconut butter

5 tablespoons (80 g/2.8 oz) light tahini

2 teaspoons (5 g) cinnamon

1 teaspoon vanilla powder or 1 tablespoon (15 ml) unsweetened vanilla extract

¼ teaspoon salt

① Preheat the oven to 285°F (140°C) fan assisted or 320°F (160°C) conventional. Line a baking tray with parchment.

② Place the macadamias and pecans on the baking tray, transfer to the oven, and bake for about 30 minutes. Remove the nuts from the oven, let cool for about 10 minutes, and then transfer to a food processor while still warm.

③ Add the remaining ingredients. Blend until smooth and creamy, 2 to 3 minutes, scraping down the sides as needed with a spatula. Transfer to a jar and store at room temperature for up to 1 week or in the fridge for up to 1 month.

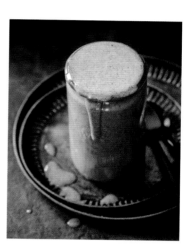

NUTRITION FACTS PER SERVING (2 TABLESPOONS/32 G/1.1 OZ):

Total carbs: 5.6 g	Fat: 21.0 g (of which saturated: 6.0 g)	SAT / MUFA / PUFA (%): 29, 55, 16
Fiber: 3.5 g	Calories: 208 kcal	Omega-6: 2.4 g. Remember, tahini breaks the omega-6 rule because of its lignan antioxidants!
Net Carbs: 2.1 g	Macronutrient ratio: Calories from carbs (4%), protein (6%), fat (90%)	
Protein: 2.9 g		

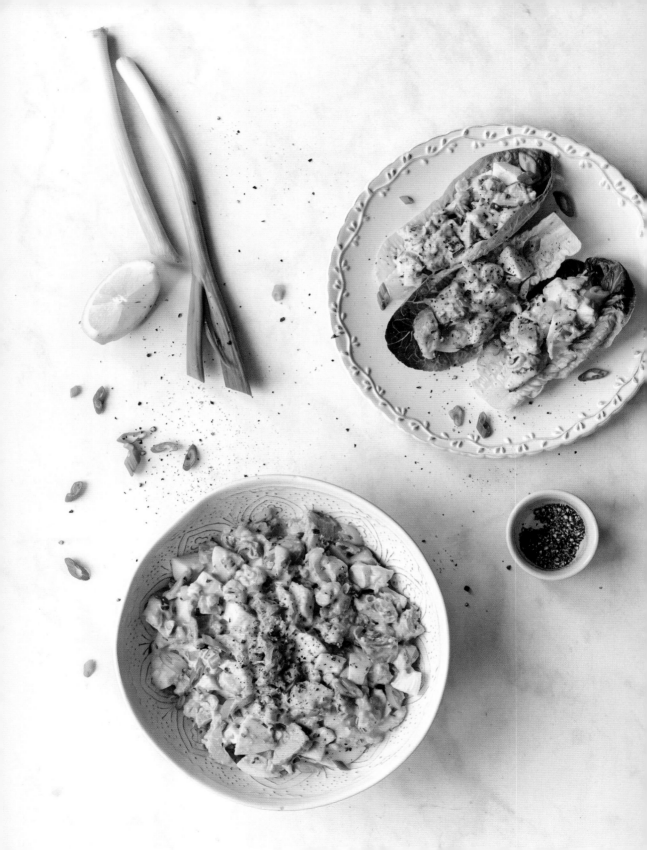

CHAPTER 4

SALADS & SOUPS

SERVINGS:
4 (sides)

HANDS-ON TIME:
10 minutes

OVERALL TIME:
10 minutes

TAVERNA-STYLE GREEK SALAD

(CONTRIBUTOR: AMY BERGER)

The recipe for this crunchy, colorful *choriatiki*—the traditional Greek name for what we English-speakers simply call "Greek salad"—was contributed by Amy Berger, a U.S. Air Force veteran, certified nutrition specialist, and the author of two best-selling books on the benefits of following a ketogenic diet. Amy says, "I eat this salad often. It's easy to make and presses all the right buttons: creamy and fatty, acidic, bitter, salty, and crunchy!" We agree. It's perfect as a summery side dish for a simple roast chicken, and as a light, warm-weather lunch.

4 to 5 (400 g/14.1 oz) medium tomatoes, roughly chopped

1 large (300 g/10.6 oz) cucumber, peeled and roughly chopped

1 medium (120 g/4.2 oz) green bell pepper, sliced

1 small (60 g/2.1 oz) red onion, sliced

16 pitted (48 g/1.7 oz) Kalamata olives

¼ cup (35 g/1.2 oz) capers, or more olives

1 teaspoon dried oregano or fresh herbs of your choice, such as parsley, cilantro, chives, or basil, divided

½ cup (120 ml) extra-virgin olive oil, divided

1 pack (200 g/7 oz) feta cheese

Optional: salt, pepper, and fresh oregano, for garnish

① Place the vegetables in a large serving bowl. Add the olives, capers, feta, half of the dried oregano and half of the olive oil. Mix to combine. Place the whole piece of feta cheese on top, sprinkle with the remaining dried oregano, and drizzle with the remaining olive oil. Season to taste and serve immediately, or store in the fridge for up to 1 day.

 FUN FACT

A landmark 2018 study published out of Harvard found that trading calories from carbs for calories from fats increases the number of calories the body burns. In the study, limiting carb intake to 20 percent of overall daily calories caused participants to burn over 200 *more* calories than when 60 percent of overall calorie intake came from carbs. (Only 7 percent of the calories in this dish come from carbs!)

NUTRITION FACTS PER SERVING (ABOUT 2 CUPS/320 G/12 OZ):

Total carbs: 11.3 g	Fat: 41.3 g (of which saturated: 12.6)	Saturated / MUFA / PUFA (%): 31, 61, 8
Fiber: 3.3 g	Calories: 443 kcal	Omega-6: 3.1 g
Net Carbs: 8 g	Macronutrient ratio: Calories from carbs (7%), protein (8%), fat (85%)	
Protein: 9.3 g		

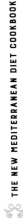

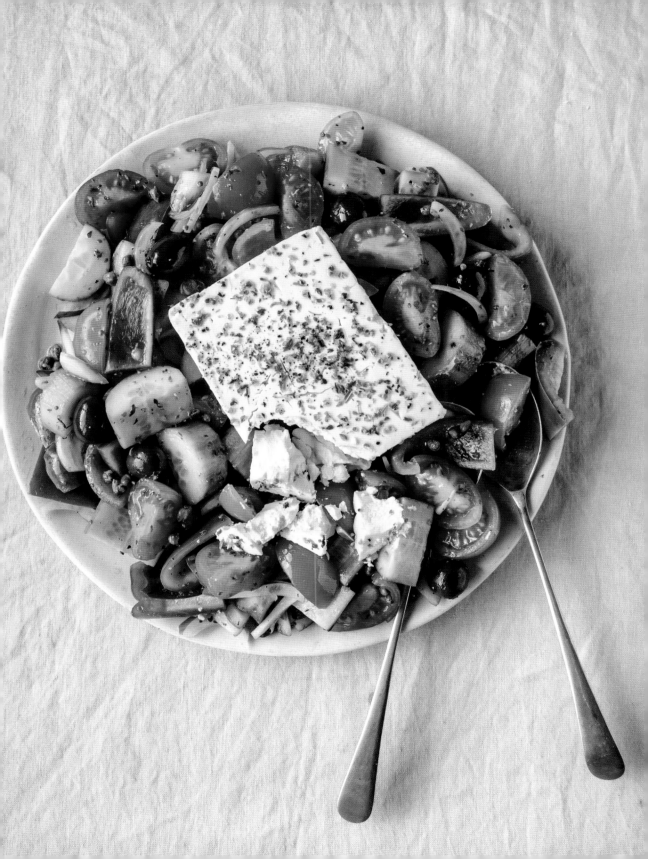

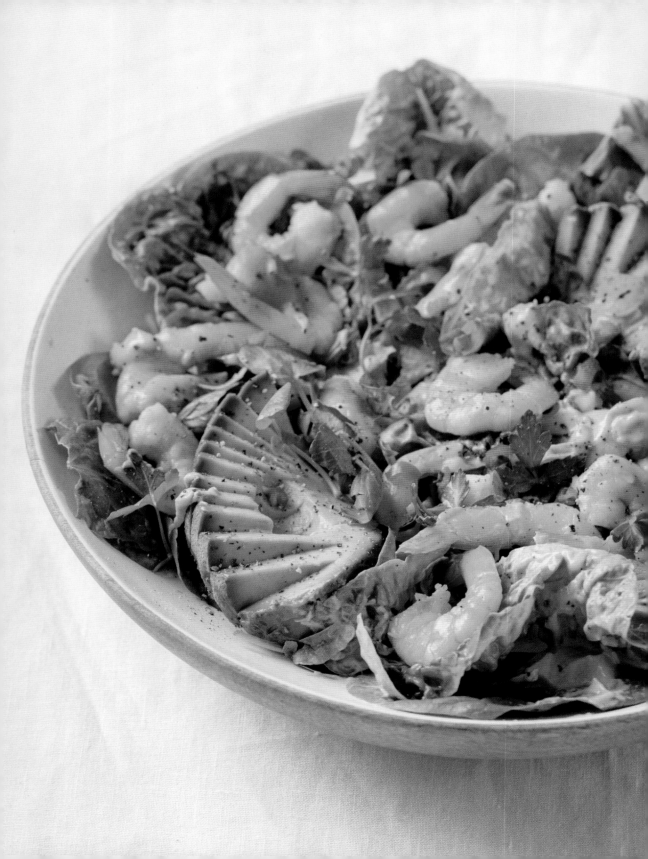

UPGRADED SHRIMP COCKTAIL SALAD

(CONTRIBUTOR: FRANZISKA SPRITZLER)

Franziska Spritzler, a registered dietitian and certified diabetes educator, gave this 1960s classic a modern makeover. Franziska, who takes a low-carb, whole-foods approach to optimal health and graceful aging, has held on to the high-protein shrimp, but banished the bland Marie-Rose sauce in favor of a thick, golden, aioli-based topping. She's also added extra greens and more healthy fats in the form of sliced avocado. The result: a quick, elegant meal for two that can be thrown together in, quite literally, minutes.

GOLDEN AIOLI

⅓ cup (80 ml) Blender Mayonnaise (page 199) or avocado oil mayonnaise

1 clove garlic, minced

1½ teaspoons unsweetened tomato purée

¼ teaspoon ground turmeric

⅛ teaspoon black pepper

SALAD

1 small (100 g/3.5 oz) gem lettuce

2 cups (60 g/2.1 oz) mixed greens: arugula, spinach, and/or watercress

7 ounces (200 g) cooked prawns or shrimp

1 medium (150 g/5.3 oz) avocado, sliced

Fresh parsley, cilantro, or chives, to garnish

Optional: 1 teaspoon chopped red chile pepper; salt and black pepper, to taste

2 to 4 lemon wedges, to serve

① To make the golden aioli: Simply combine all the ingredients in a small bowl.

② To assemble the salad: Divide the lettuce and greens between two serving bowls. Top with the prawns, avocado, and prepared aioli. Garnish with fresh herbs, season to taste, and serve immediately with the lemon wedges. Store the aioli in a sealed jar in the fridge for up to 5 days.

❈ FUN FACT ❈

Shrimp may be high in cholesterol, but that's nothing to worry about. Cholesterol is an essential molecule needed to build hormones, bile acids, cell membranes, the outsides of nerves, and even the brain itself! Cholesterol-carrying particles only become dangerous when damaged by sugar or oxidization. If you follow a low-carb lifestyle and avoid processed vegetable oils, cholesterol is actually one of the good guys!

NUTRITION FACTS PER SERVING:

Total carbs: 11.4 g

Fiber: 6.3 g

Net Carbs: 5.1 g

Protein: 23.4 g

Fat: 43.5 g (of which saturated: 6.3 g)

Calories: 516 kcal

Macronutrient ratio: Calories from carbs (4%), protein (18%), fat (78%)

Saturated / MUFA / PUFA (%): 14, 72, 14

Omega-6: 5.0 g (or 2.0 g, if you make your Blender Mayonnaise with macadamia oil)

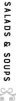

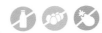
THE BEST SALMON & AVOCADO SALAD

(CONTRIBUTOR: DR. ADRIAN SOTO)

With four out of seven superfoods in a single bowl, this salad really earns its superlative! We have Dr. Adrian Soto, an M.D. and Oxford-trained Ph.D. with an expertise in ketone metabolism and diabetes, to thank for it. His recipe is a tribute to the weekly "nerd-out" dinners he and Dr. Nick Norwitz treated themselves to while studying ketones for their Ph.D.s: every single week for years, the two best friends met for dinner, and both ordered salmon and avocado salads. They couldn't have made a better choice to support their hard working brains!

POACHED SALMON

2 sprigs parsley

2 sprigs dill

1 bay leaf

2 tablespoons (30 ml) apple cider vinegar or white wine vinegar

3 whole black peppercorns

½ teaspoon salt

1 large or 2 small fillets (200 g/7 oz) wild salmon

PESTO DRESSING

2 tablespoons (30 ml) Macadamia Basil Pesto (or any pesto from pages 198 to 199)

2 tablespoons (30 ml) extra-virgin olive oil

TO ASSEMBLE

2 cups (60 g/2.1 oz) dark leafy greens, such as arugula, spinach, and/or watercress

1 medium (200 g/7 oz) zucchini, spiralized, core chopped

1 medium (150 g/5.3 oz) avocado, sliced

2 tablespoons (17 g/0.6 oz) capers, or 4 to 8 pitted olives

2 to 4 lemon wedges, to serve

① To poach the salmon: Fill a small saucepan with about 2 cups (480 ml) water (this should be just enough to cover the salmon). Add the parsley, dill, bay leaf, vinegar, peppercorns, and salt. Bring to a boil, then simmer over medium-high heat for about 10 minutes to infuse the water with flavor. Reduce the heat to medium-low and add the salmon. Cook for 5 to 6 minutes (the thicker the fillet, the longer the cooking time will be). Remove from the heat. Use a slotted spoon to transfer the salmon to a chopping board. Once it is cool enough to handle, flake the flesh and discard the skin.

② To make the pesto dressing: In a small bowl, combine the pesto and olive oil. Set aside.

③ To assemble the salad: Place the greens in a serving bowl and top them with the spiralized and chopped zucchini. (Zucchini noodles can be eaten raw: optionally, you can cook them in a pan greased with a teaspoon of avocado oil for 2 to 3 minutes.) Top with the flaked salmon flesh and avocado. Sprinkle over the capers and drizzle with the pesto dressing. Serve with lemon wedges. This salad can be stored in the fridge for up to 1 day.

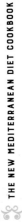

NUTRITION FACTS PER SERVING:

Total carbs: 12.1 g	Fat: 41.3 g (of which saturated: 5.9 g)	Saturated / MUFA / PUFA (%): 14, 74, 12
Fiber: 7.1 g	Calories: 499 kcal	Omega-6/3 ratio: 1.3 ☺
Net Carbs: 5 g	Macronutrient ratio: Calories from carbs (4%), protein (20%), fat (76%)	
Protein: 24 g		

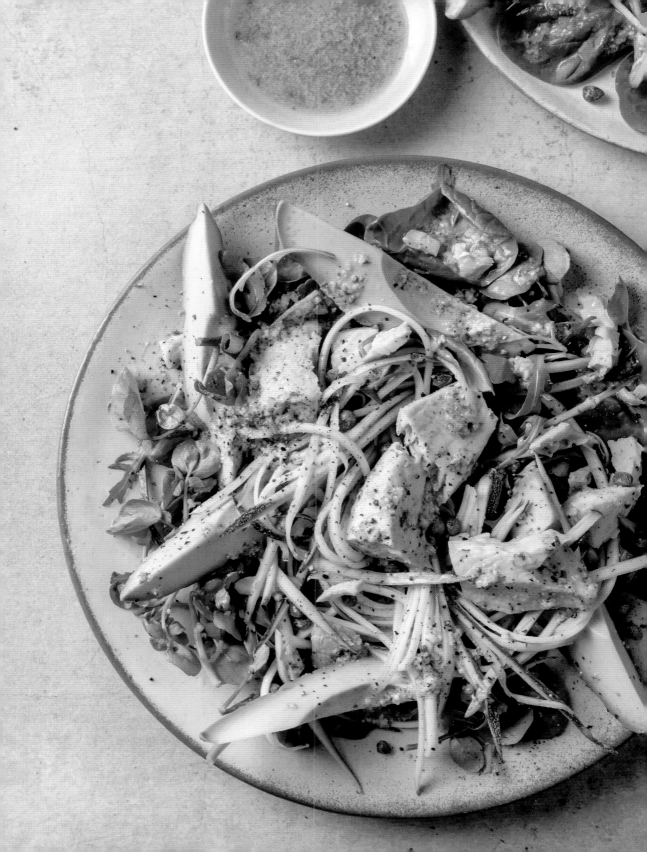

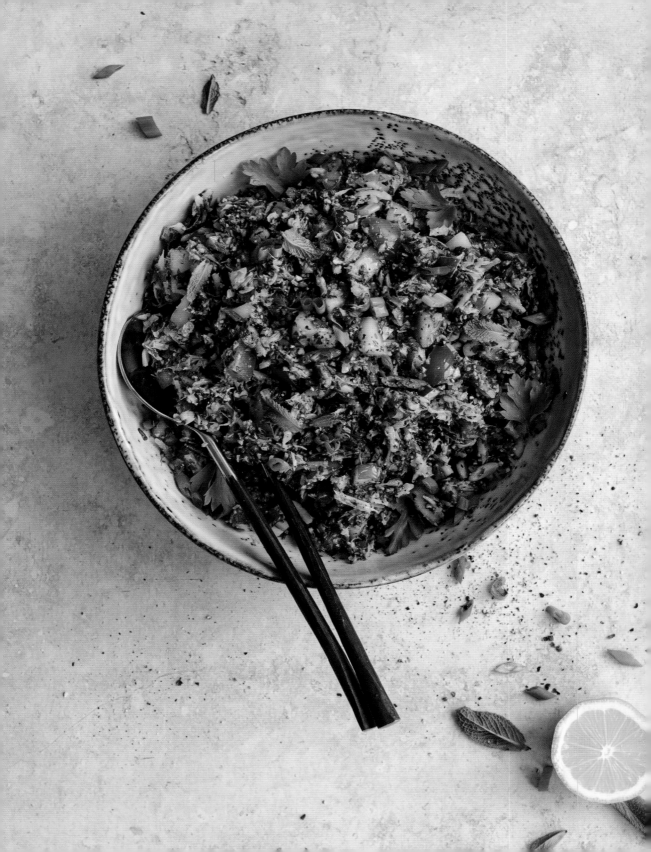

SUPERGREEN TABBOULEH

Traditionally made with bulgur wheat and a ton of fragrant herbs, classic Middle Eastern tabbouleh isn't right for a ketogenic diet. But our version, which is made with broccoli "rice," trades in the carbs for extra nutrition and top-quality fats (thanks, macadamias and EVOO!). Plus, it's just as flavorful, and it's fantastic alongside lamb, fish, and chicken dishes.

1 medium (400 g/14.1 oz) broccoli, cut into florets

2 tablespoons (30 ml) extra-virgin avocado oil or ghee

2 medium (30 g/1.1 oz) spring onions, sliced

1 small (60 g/2.1 oz) red onion, chopped

1 clove garlic, minced

1½ cups (90 g/3.2 oz) chopped fresh parsley

¾ cup (40 g/1.4 oz) chopped fresh mint

1 medium (100 g/3.5 oz) tomato, diced

1 small (150 g/5.3 oz) cucumber, peeled and diced

½ cup (120 ml) extra-virgin olive oil

½ cup (120 ml) fresh lemon juice

Salt and black pepper, to taste

¾ cup (85 g/3 oz) macadamia nuts or hazelnuts, crushed

① Place the broccoli florets in a food processor and process using a grating blade or an S blade until it resembles rice.

② Heat a large pan greased with the avocado oil over medium-high heat. Add the broccoli rice and cook for about 5 minutes. Remove from the heat and set aside to cool.

③ To the bowl with the cooked broccoli rice, add the spring onions, red onion, garlic, parsley, mint, tomato, and cucumber.

④ In a small bowl, whisk the olive oil with the lemon juice until it thickens slightly. Pour over the vegetables, stir to combine, and season with salt and pepper to taste. Top with the crushed nuts. Serve immediately or store in a sealed container in the fridge for up to 4 days.

· · · · · · · · **FUN FACT** · · · · · · · ·

This recipe may be vegetarian, but we don't promote abstaining from nutrient-rich animal foods. Interestingly, acetyl-l-carnitine levels (which you get from animal foods) tend to be lower in the brains of patients with depression, and supplementation with this nutrient, in multiple randomized controlled trials, has been shown to be as effective at relieving depression as antidepressants.

NUTRITION FACTS PER SERVING (ABOUT ¾ CUP/142 G/5 OZ):

Total carbs: 9.5 g	Fat: 25.5 g (of which saturated: 3.6 g)	Saturated / MUFA / PUFA (%): 14, 77, 9
Fiber: 3.6 g	Calories: 265 kcal	Omega-6: 2.0 g
Net Carbs: 5.9 g	Macronutrient ratio: Calories from carbs (9%), protein (5%), fat (86%)	
Protein: 3.3 g		

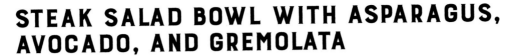

STEAK SALAD BOWL WITH ASPARAGUS, AVOCADO, AND GREMOLATA

Juicy steak and panfried asparagus feels indulgent—and it is!—but it's also a healthy, low-carb choice. Strewn with a lemony Italian gremolata sauce, which is a classic partner for beef, this colorful steak salad bowl is hearty enough to serve as a full meal for lunch or dinner.

SALAD

2 lean beef steaks (300 g/10.6 oz) such as rump, fillet, sirloin, flank, or skirt

2 tablespoons (30 ml) extra-virgin avocado oil or ghee

Salt and black pepper, to taste

14 to 16 asparagus spears (150 g/5.3 oz), hard ends snapped off

3 cups (90 g/3.2 oz) dark leafy greens, such as arugula, spinach, and/or watercress

½ small red onion (30 g/1.1 oz), sliced

½ large avocado (100 g/3.5 oz), sliced

½ recipe Gremolata (about 120 ml/½ cup)

Optional: ¼ cup (28 g/1 oz) Pecorino Romano shavings

GREMOLATA

1 bunch (60 g/2.1 oz) fresh parsley, roughly chopped

4 cloves garlic, minced

2 tablespoons (12 g/0.4 oz) finely grated lemon zest

1 tablespoon (15 ml) fresh lemon juice

½ cup (120 ml) extra-virgin olive oil

Salt and black pepper, to taste

① To make the salad: Bring the steaks to room temperature by leaving them out on the kitchen counter for 10 to 15 minutes.

② Meanwhile, prepare the gremolata: Place all of the ingredients in a food processor. Process for a few seconds until the desired consistency is reached (smooth or chunky). You will only need half of the gremolata for this recipe. Any leftover gremolata can be stored in a sealed jar in the fridge for up to 1 week.

③ Grease both sides of the steaks with 1 tablespoon (15 ml) of the avocado oil, and season with salt and pepper. Fry in a hot dry pan over high heat for 2 to 4 minutes on each side to seal in the juices. When you see the edges start to brown, it's time to flip the steaks over. Reduce the heat to medium. Continue to cook for 4 minutes (rare), 7 minutes (medium), or 11 minutes (well done). Remove the steaks from the pan and allow them to rest in a warm place for a few minutes. Slice just before serving.

④ Grease the pan where you cooked the steak with the remaining 1 tablespoon (15 ml) avocado oil. Add the asparagus spears and cook over medium heat until crisp-tender. If the asparagus spears are thick, reduce the heat to medium-low and cover with a lid. Once cooked, remove from the heat.

⑤ Divide the salad greens and sliced onion between two serving bowls. Add the sliced steak, cooked asparagus, and avocado. Top each bowl with ¼ cup (60 ml) gremolata or serve on the side. Optionally, sprinkle with the cheese. Eat warm.

NUTRITION FACTS PER SERVING:

Total carbs: 12.4 g	Fat: 65.4 g (of which saturated: 13.2 g)	Saturated / MUFA / PUFA (%): 20, 69, 11
Fiber: 6.7 g	Calories: 768 kcal	Omega-6: 7.0 g
Net Carbs: 5.7 g	Macronutrient ratio: Calories from carbs (3%), protein (19%), fat (78%)	
Protein: 35.8 g		

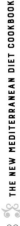

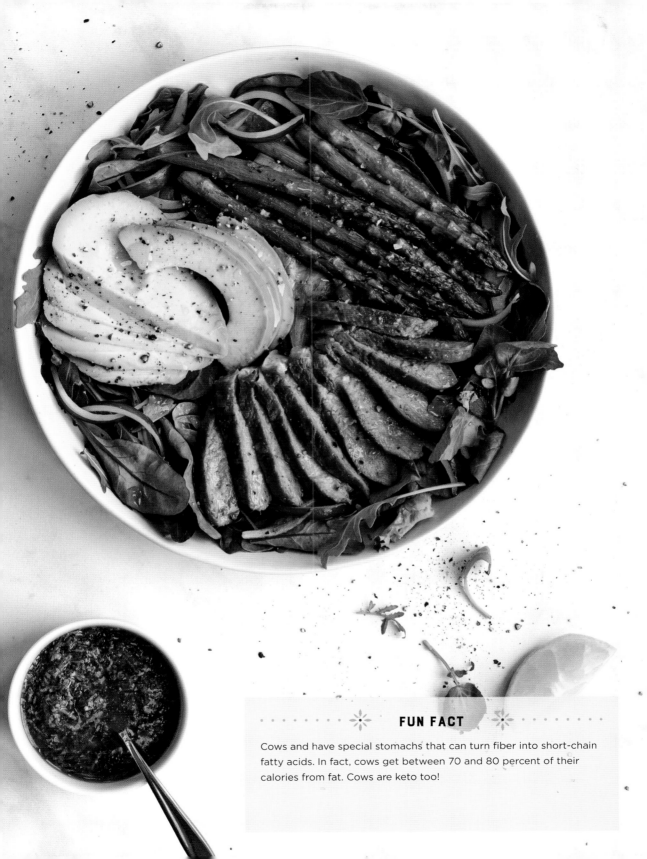

COD LIVER & EGG SALAD

(CONTRIBUTOR: ANDREW SCARBOROUGH)

This omega-3-laden masterpiece was contributed by Andrew Scarborough. When Andrew was a nutritional therapy student, he was diagnosed with a malignant brain tumor, which caused him to suffer from debilitating seizures. Surgery and chemotherapy failed, so Andrew expanded his field of study to cancer biology. He developed his own ketogenic diet, which includes lots of omega-3-rich seafood and organ meats. (Cod livers are both!) Andrew says, "My special ketogenic diet was a success and I gained back my independence." A decade later, Andrew is thriving as a student, neuroscientist, and passionate nutritional advocate. We advocate saving the drained cod oil to drizzle over cooked eggs for extra vitamins A and D and omega-3.

DRESSING

⅓ cup (80 ml) Blender Mayonnaise (page 199)

1 teaspoon Dijon or yellow mustard

Salt and black pepper, to taste

SALAD

6 large hard-boiled eggs, peeled and chopped

2 cans (200 g/7 oz) smoked cod livers, drained and chopped

1 medium (60 g/2.1 oz) celery stalk, diced

4 medium (60 g/2.1 oz) spring onions, sliced

2 tablespoons (8 g/0.3 oz) chopped fresh parsley

1 medium (150 g/5.3 oz) avocado, diced

1 head (100 g/3.5 oz) baby gem lettuce

① To make the dressing: Combine the dressing ingredients in a small bowl and set aside.

② To make the salad: Place everything apart from the lettuce in a bowl, including the dressing. Mix to combine and serve on top of crunchy lettuce leaves. The salad can be stored in a sealed jar in the fridge for up to 4 days.

 FUN FACT

Ketogenic diets have been used to treat epilepsy and seizures for more than a century. It also makes sense to apply ketogenic diets to cancer: Many tumors are carboholics due to the Warburg effect, so a low-carb diet may help suppress them. Plus, ketone supplements have been shown to treat cancer in mice, suggesting other anti-cancer keto mechanisms are at play.

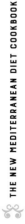

NUTRITION FACTS PER SERVING (ABOUT 170 G/6 OZ • LETTUCE LEAVES):

Total carbs: 7.5 g	Fat: 48.5 g (of which saturated: 8.9 g)	Saturated / MUFA / PUFA (%): 18, 61, 21
Fiber: 3.5 g	Calories: 495 kcal	Omega-6/3 ratio: 0.5 ☺
Net Carbs: 4 g	Macronutrient ratio: Calories from carbs (3%), protein (12%), fat (85%)	
Protein: 15.2 g		

GREEN GODDESS SALAD

The famous Green Goddess salad dressing is around a century old: It originated in San Francisco in the 1920s, and it's still one of the most popular ways to dress a summer salad. Just about everything tastes better drizzled with this herby, zingy, creamy green sauce!

GREEN GODDESS DRESSING

½ cup (120 ml) Blender Mayonnaise (page 199) or avocado oil mayonnaise

½ cup (20 g/0.7 oz) roughly chopped fresh herbs, such as parsley, dill, basil, tarragon, and/or chives

½ teaspoon onion powder

2 small (8 g/0.3 oz) canned anchovies, chopped

1 clove garlic, minced

2 tablespoons (15 ml) fresh lemon or lime juice

Salt and black pepper, to taste

SALAD

2 cups (60 g/2.1 oz) fresh spinach

2 cups (60 g/2.1 oz) watercress and/or arugula

1 small (60 g/2.1 oz) red onion, sliced

1 medium (120 g/4.2 oz) red bell pepper, sliced

1 large (200 g/7 oz) avocado, sliced

2 large hard-boiled eggs, halved

3 tablespoons (24 g/0.9 oz) pumpkin seeds, chopped

½ recipe (about 5 tablespoons) Green Goddess Dressing

① To make the dressing: Place all the dressing ingredients in a food processor and process until smooth and creamy. You will only need half of the dressing for this recipe. Store the remaining dressing in a sealed jar in the fridge for up to 5 days.

② To assemble the salad: Place the spinach and watercress in a mixing bowl. Add the onion, bell pepper, avocado, and eggs. Sprinkle with the pumpkin seeds and drizzle with the prepared dressing. Toss to combine and serve. To store, refrigerate the dressed salad for up to 1 day.

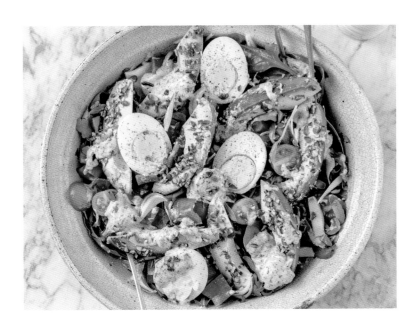

NUTRITION FACTS PER SERVING (SERVED AS A MAIN):

Total carbs: 19.6 g	Fat: 48.9 g (of which saturated: 8.1 g)	Saturated / MUFA / PUFA (%): 17, 66, 17
Fiber: 10.4 g	Calories: 556 kcal	Omega-6: 7.5 g.
Net Carbs: 9.2 g	Macronutrient ratio: Calories from carbs (7%), protein (12%), fat (81%)	
Protein: 15.7 g		

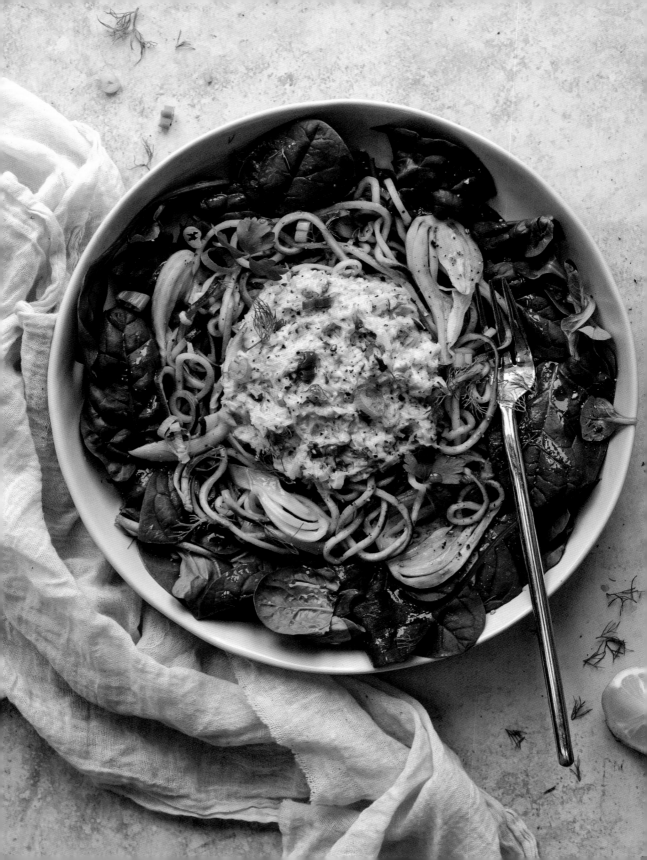

CRAB SALAD WITH FENNEL & ZUCCHINI "NOODLES"

This creamy, satisfying seafood salad is loaded with minerals, including copper, selenium, and zinc, plus a ton of prebiotic fibers to pamper the healthy microbes in your gut. True, crab might not be an inexpensive ingredient, but it's among the world's best sources of vitamin B_{12}—just half of this recipe contains 150 percent of your RDA—and its subtle flavor blends beautifully with liquoricey fennel.

CRAB TOPPING

⅓ cup (80 ml) Blender Mayonnaise (page 199) or avocado oil mayonnaise

½ teaspoon Dijon or yellow mustard

1 tablespoon (15 ml) fresh lemon juice

1 medium (15 g/0.5 oz) spring onion, sliced

1 tablespoon (4 g/1.2 oz) chopped fresh parsley, dill, or chives

7 ounces (200 g) cooked white crabmeat

Salt and black pepper, to taste

SALAD

½ small (125 g/4.4 oz) fennel bulb, sliced (fronds reserved for garnish)

1 large (250 g/8.8 oz) zucchini, spiralized

2 tablespoons (30 ml) extra-virgin avocado oil or ghee

2 cups (60 g/2.1 oz) dark leafy greens, such as arugula, watercress, spinach, or beet greens

2 tablespoons (30 ml) extra-virgin olive oil

① To make the crab topping: In a bowl, combine the mayonnaise, mustard, lemon juice, spring onion (reserve some for garnish), and herbs. Mix to combine and add the crab. Season with salt and pepper to taste.

② To make the salad: Finely slice the fennel (or use a slicing blade on your food processor) and spiralize the zucchini (or use a julienne peeler to spiralize). Place both in a hot pan greased with the avocado oil and cook for 2 to 3 minutes, until crisp-tender. Remove from the heat and set aside to cool.

③ Divide the salad greens between two serving bowls. Top each with the cooked fennel and zucchini noodles and the creamy crab filling. Drizzle with the olive oil and garnish with spring onion and/or fennel fronds. Serve immediately. The crab filling can be stored in the fridge for up to 3 days.

SALADS & SOUPS

NUTRITION FACTS PER SERVING:

Total carbs: 10.9 g

Fiber: 4 g

Net Carbs: 6.9 g

Protein: 22.8 g

Fat: 46.7 g (of which saturated: 6.4 g)

Calories: 541 kcal

Macronutrient ratio: Calories from carbs (5%), protein (17%), fat (78%)

Saturated / MUFA / PUFA (%): 14, 72, 14

Omega-6: 6.8 g

SUPERFOOD SALMON SALAD BOWL

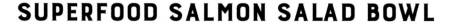

This Mediterranean superfood salad is the ultimate throw-together meal for when time is precious, but you don't want to skimp on nutrients. It's packed with omega-3 and boasts a pantheon of micronutrients, in particular vitamins A, B_6, B_{12}, C, and E, thiamin, riboflavin, niacin, folate, pantothenic acid, betaine, copper, and selenium. But that's just the tip of the iceberg. Capers, Kalamata olives, and wild Alaskan sockeye salmon also happen to be the three richest sources of the three most powerful antioxidants on the planet: quercetin, hydroxytyrosol, and astaxanthin, making this salad a real anti-inflammatory powerhouse.

SALMON

2 fillets (250 g/8.8 oz) wild salmon

Salt and black pepper, to taste

2 teaspoons (10 ml) extra-virgin avocado oil

DRESSING

1 tablespoon (9 g/0.3 oz) capers

1 teaspoon Dijon or whole-grain mustard

1 tablespoon (15 ml) apple cider vinegar or fresh lemon juice

3 tbsp (45 ml) extra-virgin olive oil

1 teaspoon coconut aminos

Salt and black pepper, to taste

SALAD

½ medium (200 g/7 oz) cucumber, diced

1 cup (50 g/1.8 oz) sugar snap peas, sliced into matchsticks

½ small (40 g/1.4 oz) red bell pepper, sliced

⅓ cup (33 g/1.2 oz) pitted Kalamata olives, halved

2 sun-dried tomatoes (14 g/0.5 oz), chopped

1 medium (150 g/5.3 oz) avocado, diced

3 tablespoons (12 g/0.4 oz) chopped fresh herbs, such as dill, chives, parsley, and/or basil

1 tablespoon (8 g/0.3 oz) pumpkin seeds

1 tablespoon (9 g/0.3 oz) sunflower seeds

① To make the salmon: Season the salmon with salt and pepper. Heat a pan greased with the avocado oil over medium heat. Add the salmon, skin-side down, and cook for 4 to 5 minutes. Flip and cook for 1 to 2 minutes or until cooked through. Remove from the heat and transfer to a plate to cool. Remove the skin from the salmon and flake into chunks.

② To make the dressing: Mix all the dressing ingredients together in a small bowl. Set aside.

③ To make the salad: Place the cucumber, sugar snap peas, bell pepper, olives, sun-dried tomatoes, avocado, and herbs in a mixing bowl, and combine well. Add the flaked salmon. Dry-fry the seeds in a pan placed over medium-low heat until lightly golden. Allow to cool, then add to the bowl. Drizzle with the prepared dressing and serve. This salad can be stored in the fridge for up to 1 day.

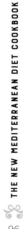

NUTRITION FACTS PER SERVING:

Total carbs: 17.6 g	Fat: 53.6 g (of which saturated: 7.8 g)	SAT / MUFA / PUFA (%): 15 / 71 / 14
Fiber: 8.6 g	Calories: 660 kcal	Omega-6/3 ratio: 1.8 ☺
Net Carbs: 9 g	Macronutrient ratio: Calories from carbs (6%), protein (19%), fat (75%)	
Protein: 31 g		

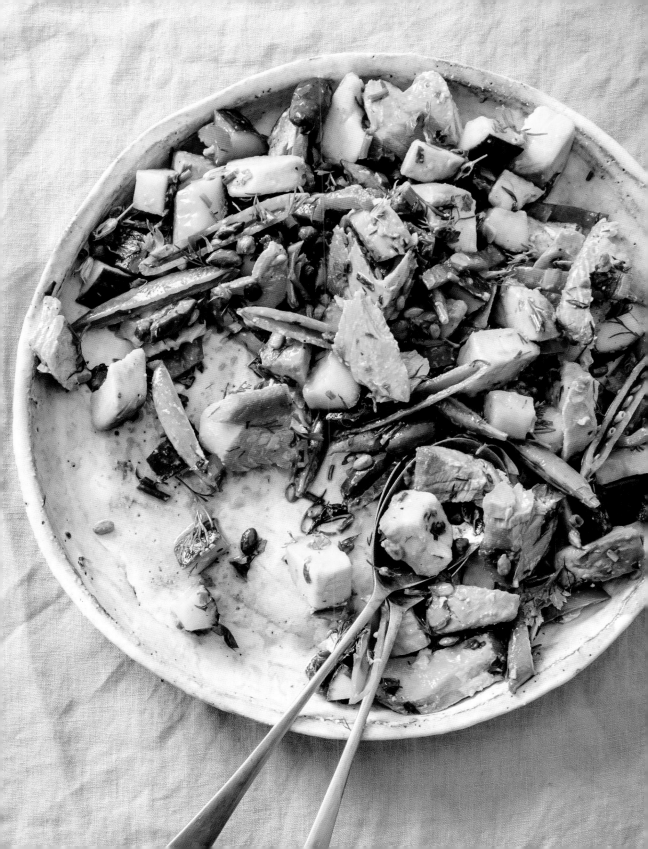

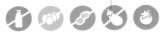

SERVINGS:	HANDS-ON TIME:	OVERALL TIME:
6	15 minutes	15 minutes

CHILLED AVOCADO PESTO SOUP

MUFA-rich avocados aren't just for salads and sandwiches: you can also use them to make velvety chilled soups like this one. Spiked with fresh citrus juice and homemade jalapeño mint pesto, it's so refreshing on a hot summer afternoon, especially as a light lunch or an appetizer—and the recipe makes enough to feed a small crowd, too.

SOUP

2 large (400 g/14.1 oz) avocados, pitted and peeled

1 large (300 g/10.6 oz) cucumber, peeled and roughly chopped

2 cloves garlic, crushed

¼ cup (60 ml) fresh lime or lemon juice

2½ cups (600 ml) vegetable or chicken stock

1 cup (240 ml) coconut milk

Salt and black pepper, to taste

¾ cup (180 ml) Jalapeño Mint Pesto or other pesto on pages 198 to 199, about 2 tablespoons (30 ml) per serving

¼ cup (15 g/0.5 oz) chopped fresh chives or spring onion

Optional: crumbled feta or goat's cheese, to serve

Focaccia (page 179), to serve

① To make the soup: Place all the ingredients except the pesto, chives, and optional cheese in a blender. Process until smooth. Divide among serving bowls, top each with chives, and drizzle with 2 tablespoons (30 g) pesto.

② Refrigerate (without toppings) in a sealed container for up to 3 days. Optionally, top with crumbled feta. Serve with a slice of focaccia!

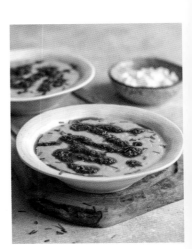

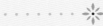 **FUN FACT**

Warning: This Fun Fact gets a PG-13 rating! Avocados are also called alligator pears or butter pears. Why the euphemism? Well, I bet you didn't know that "avocado" is derived from the Aztec word *āhuacatl*, which means testicle. Seems avocados really do grow in pairs.

NUTRITION FACTS PER SERVING (ABOUT 1¼ CUPS/300 ML):

Total carbs: 11.9 g	Fat: 42.3 g (of which saturated: 14.1 g)	Saturated / MUFA / PUFA (%): 33, 60, 7
Fiber: 5.9 g	Calories: 421 kcal	Omega-6: 2.75 g
Net Carbs: 6 g	Macronutrient ratio: Calories from carbs (6%), protein (4%), fat (90%)	
Protein: 4.1 g		

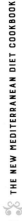

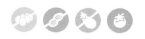

CAULIFLOWER & BLUE CHEESE SOUP

(CONTRIBUTOR: PROFESSOR KIERAN CLARKE)

A strong blue cheese like Roquefort can really stand up to cauliflower's sulfurous kick, so you can't do better than to pair them in a creamy, starch-free soup. The recipe for this one was contributed by Professor Kieran Clarke of Oxford University, a world-renowned expert in ketone science, whose work has shown that ketones can increase the efficiency of a working heart by 25 percent, and that sugar and typical high-carb Western diets worsen brain network stability, a marker of brain aging, while ketones and ketogenic diets improve it! Kieran recommends that you have yours with a healthy slice of focaccia (page 179)!

2 tablespoons (30 ml) extra-virgin avocado oil

1 small (60 g/2.1 oz) red onion, diced

1 medium (60 g/2.1 oz) celery stalk, sliced

1 medium (500 g/1.1 lb) cauliflower, cut into small florets

2 cups (480 ml) vegetable or chicken stock

¼ cup (60 ml) goat's cream or heavy whipping cream

Salt and black pepper, to taste

1 cup (113 g/4 oz) crumbled goat's or sheep's blue cheese, such as Roquefort

2 tablespoons (6 g/0.2 oz) chopped fresh chives

5 tablespoons (75 ml) extra-virgin olive oil

① Heat a medium saucepan greased with the avocado oil over medium heat. Sweat the onion and celery for 3 to 5 minutes, until soft and fragrant. Add the cauliflower florets and cook for 5 minutes. Add the vegetable stock and bring to a boil. Cook for about 10 minutes, or until the cauliflower is tender. Remove from the heat and let cool for a few minutes.

② Add the cream. Use an immersion blender, or pour into a blender, to process until smooth and creamy. Season with salt and pepper to taste. Divide the soup between serving bowls and top with the crumbled blue cheese, chives, and olive oil. To store, let cool and refrigerate in a sealed container for up to 5 days.

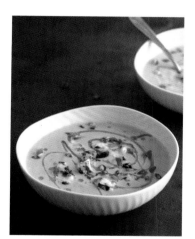

NUTRITION FACTS PER SERVING (ABOUT 1 CUP/240 ML):

Total carbs: 7.9 g	Fat: 35.2 g (of which saturated: 12.6 g)	Saturated / MUFA / PUFA (%): 36, 56, 8
Fiber: 2.6 g	Calories: 372 kcal	Omega-6: 2.2 g
Net Carbs: 5.3 g	Macronutrient ratio: Calories from carbs (6%), protein (8%), fat (86%)	
Protein: 7.8 g		

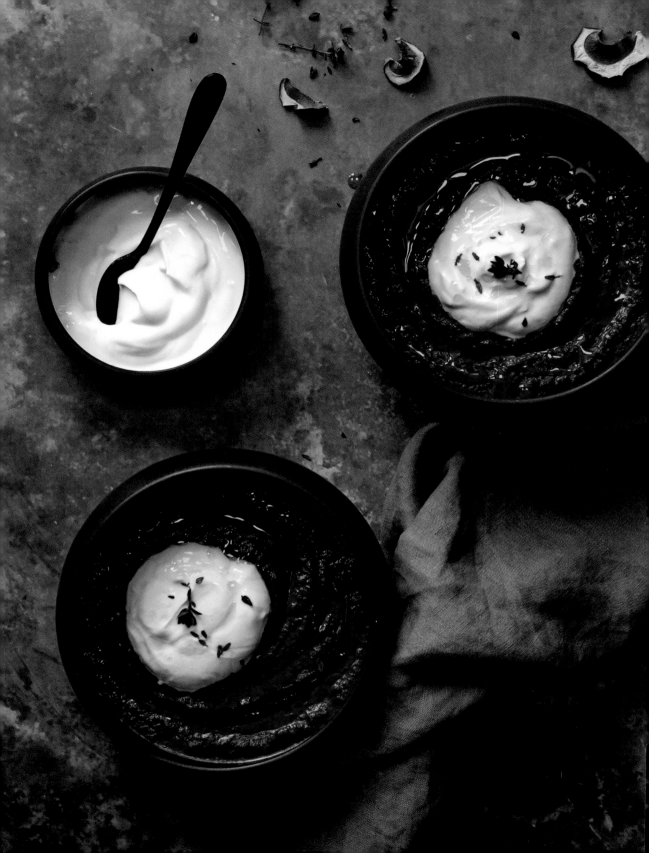

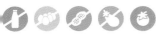

CREAMY WILD MUSHROOM SOUP

This soup is rich and creamy with earthy flavor from porcini mushrooms, caramelized flavor from roasted cauliflower, and finished with a drizzle of extra-virgin olive oil. Just what you need for a chilly fall evening!

1 cup (30 g/1.1 oz) dried porcini mushrooms and/or morel mushrooms

2 cups (480 ml) boiling water, for soaking the mushrooms

½ medium (350 g/12.4 oz) cauliflower, cut into florets and sliced

1 small (60 g/2.1 oz) red onion, roughly chopped

2 cloves garlic, halved

¼ cup (60 ml) extra-virgin avocado oil or ghee

3 cups (720 ml) chicken stock, bone broth, or vegetable stock (plus more if needed)

12 ounces (340 g) brown mushrooms or other fresh mushrooms of your choice, sliced

Few sprigs fresh thyme, leaves only, or 1 teaspoon dried thyme

1 cup (240 ml) coconut cream, goat's cream, or heavy whipping cream

½ cup (120 ml) extra-virgin olive oil, to drizzle

Fresh thyme sprigs, to serve

Optional: sour cream, coconut yogurt, or coconut cream, to serve

1) Place the dried mushrooms in a small bowl and pour over enough boiling water to cover them. Set aside to soak for about 30 minutes. Preheat the oven to 355°F (180°C) fan assisted or 400°F (200°C) conventional.

2) Place the cauliflower florets, onion, and garlic on a baking tray. Drizzle with the avocado oil or ghee and bake for about 30 minutes. Remove from the oven and set aside.

3) Meanwhile, pour the chicken stock into a large pot and bring to a boil. Add the cauliflower mixture, soaked porcini mushrooms (including the soaking liquid), and fresh mushrooms. Cook for about 8 minutes, until the mushrooms are tender. Add the thyme and coconut cream and heat through. Remove from the heat and set aside to cool for a few minutes.

4) Use an immersion blender, or pour into a blender, to process until smooth and creamy. If the soup is too thick, add water or more stock until the desired consistency is reached.

5) To serve, pour into serving bowls and drizzle each with the olive oil. Garnish with more thyme and serve with a dollop of sour cream, if using. To store, let cool and refrigerate in a sealed container for up to 5 days.

NUTRITION FACTS PER SERVING (ABOUT 1 CUP/240 ML):

Total carbs: 9.8 g	Fat: 32.9 g (of which saturated: 12.9 g)	Saturated / MUFA / PUFA (%): 39, 53, 8
Fiber: 2.4 g	Calories: 340 kcal	Omega-6: 2.3 g
Net Carbs: 7.4 g	Macronutrient ratio: Calories from carbs (8%), protein (6%), fat (86%)	
Protein: 5.3 g		

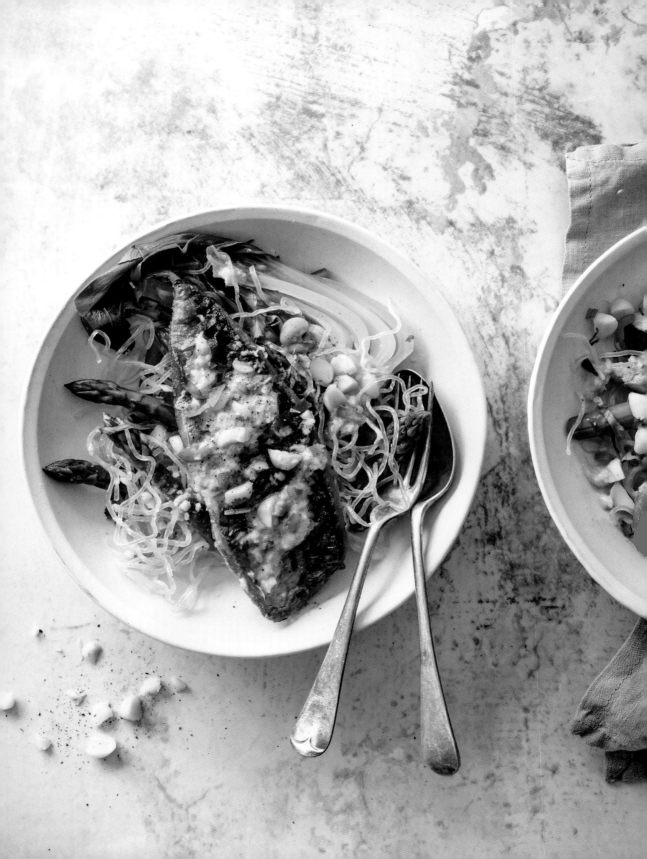

CHAPTER 5

LUNCHES

GREEK SPANAKORIZO

This one-pot spin on *spanakorizo*, or Greek spinach rice, is bursting with flavor, thanks to aromatic herbs, zingy lemon, creamy feta, and a generous drizzle of extra-virgin olive oil. If you're a particular fan of garlic, feel free to add extra: Even the National Cancer Institute recognizes garlic as one of several vegetables with anticancer properties.

1 large (1 kg/2.2 lb) cauliflower

¼ cup (60 ml) extra-virgin avocado oil

1 small (60 g/2.1 oz) red onion, diced

2 cloves garlic, minced

2 tablespoons (30 ml) fresh lemon juice

7 ounces (200 g) frozen spinach, thawed and squeezed dry, then chopped (weight excludes water squeezed out)

1 teaspoon fresh lemon zest

½ cup (30 g/1.1 oz) chopped mixed fresh herbs of your choice, such as parsley, oregano, basil, rosemary, and dill

Salt and black pepper, to taste

2 cups (300 g/10.6 oz) crumbled feta cheese

Optional: ¾ cup (75 g/2.7 oz) black olives, sliced

¼ cup (60 ml) extra-virgin olive oil

① Run the cauliflower florets through a hand grater or food processor with the S or the grating blade. Process until the florets resemble grains of rice.

② Grease a large, shallow, ovenproof saucepan or a casserole dish with the avocado oil and add the onion. Cook over medium heat for 5 minutes. Add the garlic and cook for 1 minute. Add the cauliflower rice and lemon juice and cook for 7 to 10 minutes, stirring constantly. Add the spinach, lemon zest, and herbs (optionally, reserve some herbs for garnish). Cook to heat through for just 1 to 2 minutes. Season with salt and pepper to taste.

③ Top with the crumbled feta and, optionally, olives. Place under a broiler for 3 to 5 minutes, until the feta is lightly browned. Finally, drizzle with the olive oil and serve. To store, let cool and place in a sealed container. Refrigerate for up to 5 days.

FUN FACTS

To optimize garlic's health benefits, chop it and then let it sit for 10 minutes before using it in your recipes. Chopping activates alliinase, an antioxidant and anticancer enzyme found in garlic.

Garlic may make your breath stink, but the bad mouth bacteria *Porphyromonas gingivalis* may contribute to Alzheimer's disease! Bottom line, brush your teeth, not for your breath but for your brain!

NUTRITION FACTS PER SERVING (1½ CUPS/250 G/8.8 OZ):

Total carbs: 13.8 g	Fat: 29.5 g (of which saturated: 10 g)	SAT / MUFA / PUFA (%): 34, 56, 10
Fiber: 4.8 g	Calories: 353 kcal	Omega-6: 2.3 g
Net Carbs: 9 g	Macronutrient ratio: Calories from carbs	
Protein: 11.9 g	(10%), protein (14%), fat (76%)	

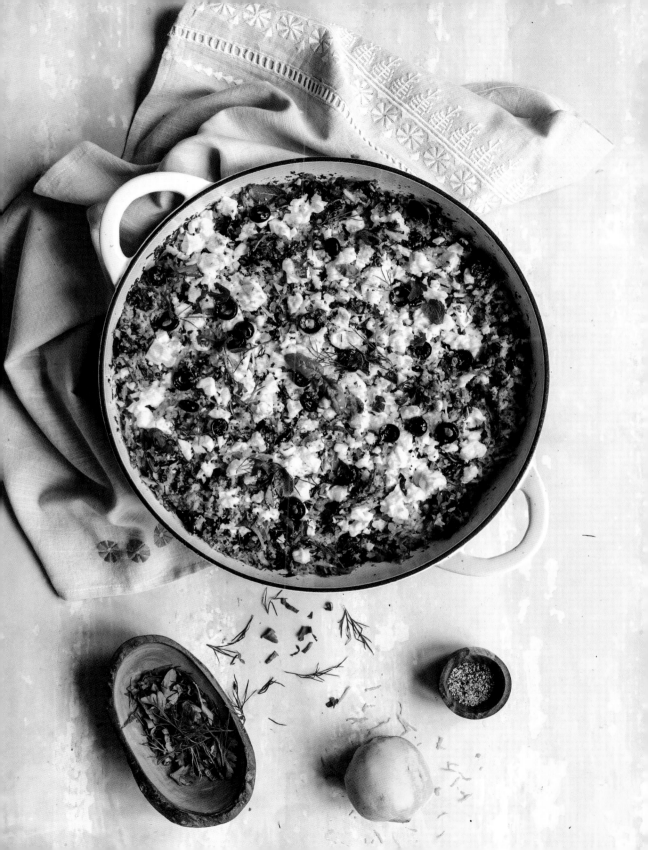

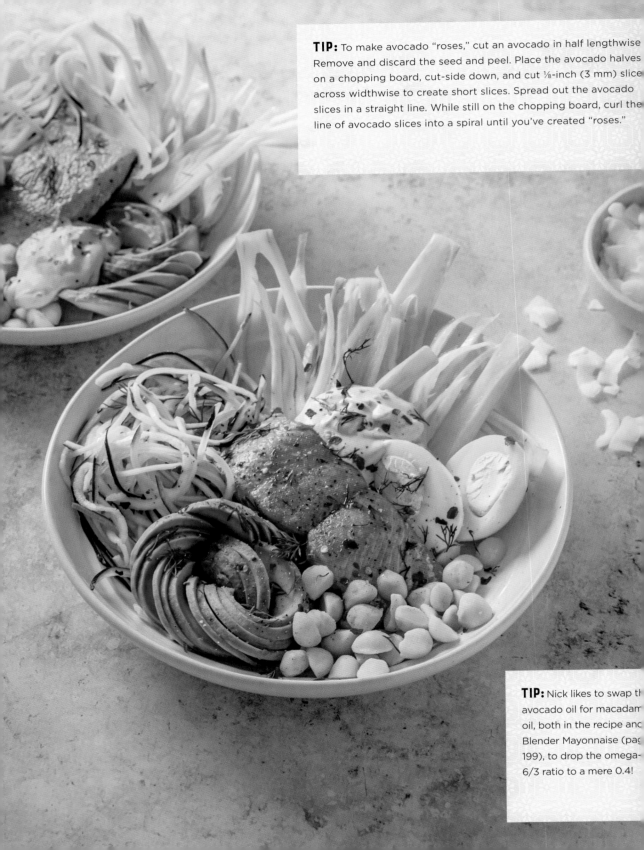

TIP: To make avocado "roses," cut an avocado in half lengthwise Remove and discard the seed and peel. Place the avocado halves on a chopping board, cut-side down, and cut ⅛-inch (3 mm) slice across widthwise to create short slices. Spread out the avocado slices in a straight line. While still on the chopping board, curl the line of avocado slices into a spiral until you've created "roses."

TIP: Nick likes to swap th avocado oil for macadam oil, both in the recipe and Blender Mayonnaise (pag 199), to drop the omega-6/3 ratio to a mere 0.4!

FIVE-SUPERFOOD SALMON BRAIN BOWL

(CONTRIBUTOR: DR. NICHOLAS NORWITZ)

This brain-boosting formula was invented by neuroscientist Dr. Nick Norwitz. Salmon contains DHA and the antioxidant astaxanthin, while avocado, zucchini, and fennel provide prebiotics that support the gut-brain axis. EVOO contains oleocanthal and hydroxytyrosol, which can prevent the buildup of Alzheimer's amyloid plaques and tau tangles.

SALMON

2 medium fillets (300 g/10.6 oz) wild salmon

2 teaspoons (10 ml) fresh lemon juice

Pink Himalayan salt and black pepper, to taste

1 tablespoon (15 ml) extra-virgin avocado oil

ZUCCHINI & FENNEL NOODLES

½ small bulb (150 g/5.3 oz) fennel bulb (fronds reserved for garnish)

1 tablespoon (15 ml) extra-virgin avocado oil or olive oil

1 medium (150 g/5.3 oz) zucchini, spiralized and core chopped

GOLDEN MAYO

¼ cup (60 ml) Blender Mayonnaise (page 199) or avocado oil mayonnaise

1 tablespoon (15 ml) Dijon or yellow mustard

¼ teaspoon ground turmeric

1 teaspoon chopped fresh tarragon or dill

TO ASSEMBLE

1 large (200 g/7 oz) avocado, sliced or shaped into "roses" (see Tip)

2 teaspoons (10 ml) fresh lemon juice

2 large hard-boiled or soft-boiled eggs, halved

½ cup (67 g/2.4 oz) macadamia nuts

Pinch of pink Himalayan salt or LoSalt, to taste

Pinch of black pepper and/or chile flakes, to taste

1 tablespoon (4 g/0.2 oz) chopped fresh dill, tarragon, or fennel fronds

Optional: ½ cup (30 g/1.1 oz) unsweetened large coconut flakes

① To make the salmon: Drizzle the salmon with the lemon juice and season with salt and pepper. Grease a pan with the avocado oil. Add the salmon and cook over medium heat for 3 to 4 minutes per side, until browned and cooked through. Remove from the pan and set aside.

② To make the noodles: Using a sharp knife, thinly slice the fennel, or process in a food processor using the slicing blade. Grease the pan you cooked the salmon in with the avocado oil and add the zucchini and fennel. Cook over medium-high heat for 2 to 3 minutes, then remove from the heat and set aside. (You can also serve the zucchini and fennel raw.)

③ To make the golden mayo: Combine all of the ingredients in a small bowl and set aside.

④ To assemble: Divide the zucchini and fennel noodles between two bowls. Add the salmon and avocado and drizzle with the lemon juice. Add the eggs and macadamias and season with salt, pepper, and chile flakes. Top with fresh herbs and serve with the golden mayo and crunchy coconut flakes on the side, if using. Store in the fridge for up to 1 day.

NUTRITION FACTS PER SERVING (1 BOWL):

Total carbs: 22.9 g	Fat: 93.9 g (of which saturated: 14.5 g)	SAT / MUFA / PUFA (%): 15, 72, 13
Fiber: 13.1 g	Calories: 1076 kcal	Omega-6/3 ratio: 1.2 ☺
Net Carbs: 9.8 g	Macronutrient ratio: Calories from carbs	
Protein: 43.3 g	(4%), protein (16%), fat (80%)	

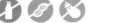

TURKEY MEATBALLS WITH SALSA VERDE

These quick-prep meatballs, served with a fragrant, herby, emerald-green salsa verde, are perfect for batch cooking and lunch boxes. Try them with an EVOO-dressed side salad for a complete meal. You'll have plenty of leftover salsa verde: it makes a great condiment for roasted or grilled meat or fish.

SALSA VERDE

1 cup (30 g/1.1 oz) packed fresh basil leaves

2 cups (50 g/1.8 oz) packed fresh parsley

¼ cup (6 g/0.2 oz) chopped fresh mint leaves

2 tablespoons (17 g/0.6 oz) capers

4 pieces (16 g/0.6 oz) canned anchovies, drained

2 cloves garlic, roughly chopped

3 tablespoons (45 ml) apple cider vinegar

2 tablespoons (30 ml) fresh lemon juice

¾ cup (180 ml) extra-virgin olive oil

Salt and black pepper, to taste

MEATBALLS

1 tablespoon (15 ml) extra-virgin avocado oil or ghee

1 small (60 g/2.1 oz) red onion, diced

1 teaspoon fresh thyme leaves

1.1 pounds (500 g) ground turkey (15% fat)

1 large egg

½ teaspoon salt

½ teaspoon black pepper

Zest from 1 organic lemon

3 tablespoons (24 g/0.9 oz) coconut flour

Serve with ½ recipe (¾ cup/180 ml) prepared Salsa Verde, about 3 tablespoons (45 ml) per serving

① To make the salsa: Place all of the ingredients in a food processor and process until smooth. (Alternatively, you can use a knife to chop the herbs, capers, anchovies, and garlic, and then mix them with the vinegar, lemon juice, and olive oil in a bowl. Season with salt and pepper.) Set aside. You will only need half of the recipe. Store the remainder in a sealed jar in the fridge for up to 2 weeks.

② To make the meatballs: Heat a skillet greased with the avocado oil over medium heat. Add the onion and thyme and cook until fragrant, about 3 minutes. Let cool slightly. Add the onion mixture to a bowl with the ground turkey, egg, salt, pepper, lemon zest, and coconut flour. Mix to combine. Use your hands to form 16 equal size (about 40 g/1.4 oz each) meatballs. Cook the meatballs in the skillet in which you cooked the onion in batches for about 8 minutes, turning once or twice to ensure they are browned on all sides.

③ Eat warm drizzled with the salsa verde and with a simple side salad or let the meatballs cool and refrigerate for up to 4 days or freeze for up to 3 months.

 FUN FACT

After Thanksgiving turkey dinner, you probably feel like fasting. Intermittent fasting has been shown, in animals, to protect against the amyloid and tau pathologies of Alzheimer's disease!

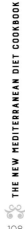
THE NEW MEDITERRANEAN DIET COOKBOOK

NUTRITION FACTS PER SERVING (4 MEATBALLS · 3 TABLESPOONS [45 ML] SALSA VERDE):

Total carbs: 4.7 g	Fat: 41.9 g (of which saturated: 8.8 g)	SAT / MUFA / PUFA (%): 21, 64, 15
Fiber: 1.9 g	Calories: 494 kcal	Omega-6: 1.8 g
Net Carbs: 2.8 g	Macronutrient ratio: Calories from carbs (2%), protein (21%), fat (77%)	
Protein: 25 g		

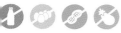

SARDINE PATTIES WITH OLIVE TAPENADE

Sardines are one of the most underestimated superfoods. Like salmon, they're full of brain- supporting DHA, and are both sustainable and inexpensive. If you're wondering what to make with canned sardines, start with this Greek-style dish: it's served with an addictive Kalamata olive tapenade that also supports brain health. Like the red onion in the sardine patties, the capers in the tapenade are a good source of quercetin, an antioxidant that inhibits the "CypA-MMP9" inflammatory pathway that contributes to blood-brain barrier breakdown and Alzheimer's disease.

SARDINE PATTIES

- 2 tablespoons (30 ml) extra-virgin avocado oil or ghee, divided
- ½ small (30 g/1.1 oz) red onion, diced
- 2 to 3 cans (285 g/10 oz drained) sardines
- Zest of 1 organic lemon
- ¼ cup (15 g/0.5 oz) chopped fresh dill or parsley
- 1 large egg
- 2 tablespoons (16 g/0.6 oz) coconut flour
- Salt and black pepper, to taste
- Lemon wedges, to serve

OLIVE TAPENADE

- ½ cup (100 g/3.5 oz) pitted and drained Kalamata olives
- 1 clove garlic, minced
- 1 tablespoon (9 g/0.3 oz) drained capers
- 2 pieces (8 g/0.3 oz) canned anchovies, drained
- 2 tablespoons (8 g/0.3 oz) chopped fresh parsley
- 1 tablespoon (15 ml) fresh lemon juice
- 3 tablespoons (45 ml) extra-virgin olive oil
- Black pepper, to taste

① To make the patties: Heat a skillet greased with 1 tablespoon (15 ml) avocado oil over medium-high heat. Cook the onion for 3 to 5 minutes, until fragrant. Remove from the heat and place in a large bowl. Add the remaining patty ingredients and mix well. Using your hands, shape into 6 medium-size fish patties (about 66 g/2.3 oz each). Refrigerate for 20 minutes.

② Grease the same pan in which you cooked the onion with the remaining 1 tablespoon (15 ml) avocado oil and cook the patties in batches for 3 minutes per side, then transfer to a paper towel–lined plate.

③ You can make the tapenade in one of two ways: Either place all the ingredients in a blender and blitz into a smooth paste, or pound all the ingredients in a mortar and pestle. This traditional method is not only therapeutic—all that pounding relieves tension!—but also produces a much better texture.

④ Serve the fish patties with the tapenade and a side salad of your choice. To store, refrigerate the cooked fish patties for up to 4 days and the tapenade in a sealed container for up to 1 week.

NUTRITION FACTS PER SERVING (2 PATTIES + ABOUT ¼ CUP [60 ML] OLIVE TAPENADE):

Total carbs: 5.3 g	Fat: 45.2 g (of which saturated: 7.5 g)	SAT / MUFA / PUFA (%): 17, 65, 18
Fiber: 2.8 g	Calories: 545 kcal	Omega-6/3 ratio: 2.0 ☺
Net Carbs: 2.5 g	Macronutrient ratio: Calories from carbs (2%), protein (21%), fat (77%)	
Protein: 28.4 g		

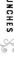

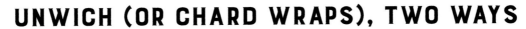

	SERVINGS:	HANDS-ON TIME:	OVERALL TIME:
	2	10 minutes	10 minutes

UNWICH (OR CHARD WRAPS), TWO WAYS

These wraps are so easy to put together. Just combine your protein of choice with your favorite vegetables and dressing, then roll them up in chard or lettuce. For the tuna niçoise version, buy skipjack tuna—skipjack are lower on the food chain and have about a third as much mercury as albacore or yellowfin. (Skipjack tuna is often labeled as "light.")

ANTIPASTI CHICKEN WRAPS

2 tablespoons (30 ml) Blender Mayonnaise (page 199) or avocado oil mayonnaise

2 tablespoons (30 ml) Macadamia Basil Pesto or any pesto on pages 198 to 199

1½ teaspoons fresh lemon juice

Salt and black pepper, to taste

1 tablespoon (4 g/0.2 oz) chopped fresh parsley or chives

6 ounces (170 g) shredded cooked chicken breast

½ medium (60 g/2.1 oz) red bell pepper, sliced

4 halves (50 g/1.8 oz) artichoke hearts, sliced

¼ small (15 g/0.5 oz) red onion, sliced

1 tablespoon (9 g/0.3 oz) capers

TUNA NIÇOISE WRAPS

3 tablespoons (45 ml) Blender Mayonnaise (page 199) or avocado oil mayonnaise

½ teaspoon Dijon or yellow mustard

1 teaspoon fresh lemon juice

Salt and black pepper, to taste

1 teaspoon chopped fresh dill

5 ounces (142 g) drained canned tuna

¼ small (15 g/0.5 oz) red onion, sliced

6 green pitted olives (20 g/0.7 oz), sliced

4 radishes (50 g/1.8 oz), sliced

2 hard-boiled eggs, chopped

6 chard leaves (120 g/4.2 oz), stems removed, or soft lettuce leaves

① To make the antipasti chicken wraps: Prepare the dressing by combining the mayo, pesto, lemon juice, salt, pepper, and parsley. Mix in the shredded chicken, bell pepper, artichoke, onion, and capers.

② To make the tuna niçoise wraps: Prepare the dressing by combining the mayonnaise, mustard, lemon juice, salt, pepper, and dill. Add the drained tuna and onion. Mix to combine. Mix in the olives, radishes, and eggs.

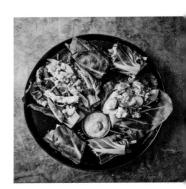

③ To assemble the wraps: Place a piece of parchment paper or aluminum foil on your work surface. Place 3 chard leaves on top in a single layer, slightly overlapping. Add the filling. Roll up the parchment paper tightly, tucking the edges as you go, like a sushi roll. Pull the parchment paper up and out as you fold it over so you're not tucking the paper into the wrap. Repeat for the second wrap. Cut the finished wraps in half with a sharp knife. To eat, simply pull the parchment paper away as you go. (1 wrap = both halves per serving.)

NUTRITION FACTS PER SERVING (1 ANTIPASTI CHICKEN/TUNA NIÇOISE WRAP):

Total carbs: 9.2/5.1 g
Fiber: 3.7/2 g
Net Carbs: 5.5/3.1 g
Protein: 27.7/21.7 g

Fat: 23.5/25.9 g (of which saturated: 3.9/4.6 g)
Calories: 371/334 kcal
Macronutrient ratio: Calories from carbs (6/4%), protein (31/26%), fat (63/70%)

SAT / MUFA / PUFA (%): 17, 72, 11 / 18, 70, 12
Omega-6: 2.1 / 2.6 g

THE NEW MEDITERRANEAN DIET COOKBOOK

110

STUFFED AVOCADOS, TWO WAYS

If you've got a ripe, fiber-rich, antioxidant-jammed avocado on hand, you've basically got an instant healthy lunch. Stuff yours with whichever low-carb fillings you have on hand: bacon and blue cheese; hard-boiled eggs, onion, and Blender Mayonnaise (page 199); or shredded beef and Pecorino Romano. We have to confess, though, that these two seafood-based versions are our favorites.

SARDINE & COD ROE

3 ounces (85 g) drained canned sardines, preferably in brine

1.5 ounces (43 g) canned cod roe

1 tablespoon (15 ml) Blender Mayonnaise (page 199) or avocado mayonnaise

1 medium (15 g/0.5 oz) spring onion, sliced

¼ teaspoon ground turmeric

1 teaspoon fresh lemon juice

¼ teaspoon black pepper

Salt, to taste

CRAB

3.5 ounces (100 g) white crabmeat

1 small (40 g/1.4 oz) celery stalk, finely sliced

1 tablespoon (4 g/0.2 oz) chopped fresh parsley or chives

¼ small (15 g/0.5 oz) red onion, diced

2 tablespoons (30 ml) Blender Mayonnaise (page 199) or avocado oil mayonnaise

1 teaspoon fresh lemon juice

¼ teaspoon Dijon or yellow mustard

Salt and black pepper, to taste

8 hazelnuts (10 g/0.4 oz), crushed, for topping

TO ASSEMBLE

1 extra-large (250 g/8.8 oz) avocado or 2 small (250 g/8.8 oz) avocados

Chopped fresh herbs, for garnish

Black pepper

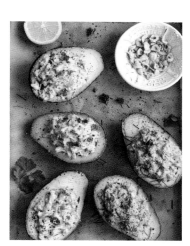

① To make the sardine & cod roe: Place the sardines in a mixing bowl. Add the drained cod roe, mayonnaise, spring onion, turmeric, lemon juice, pepper, and salt. Use a fork to mash until well combined.

② To make the crab: Place the crabmeat in a mixing bowl. Add the celery, parsley, onion, mayonnaise, lemon juice, mustard, salt, and pepper. Use a fork to combine.

③ To assemble: Leaving a ½-inch (1 cm) layer of avocado along the insides of the skins, scoop the middle of the avocado halves out, cut into small pieces, and add to the bowl with the prepared filling. Combine well.

④ Fill the avocado halves with the mixture. Garnish with the fresh herbs and black pepper. If making the crab-stuffed avocados, top with crushed hazelnuts and serve immediately.

NUTRITION FACTS PER SERVING (½ EXTRA-LARGE SARDINE AND COD ROE/CRAB AVOCADO):

Total carbs: 11.8/13.7 g

Fiber: 8.7/9.6 g

Net Carbs: 3.1/4.1 g

Protein: 15.8/13.3 g

Fat: 30.3/34.9 g (of which saturated: 4.4/4.7 g)

Calories: 367/401 kcal

Macronutrient ratio: Calories from carbs (4/4%), protein (18/14%), fat (78/82%)

SAT / MUFA / PUFA (%): 15, 63, 22 / 13, 72, 15

Sardine, Omega-6/3 ratio: 1.2 ☺

Crab, Omega-6: 1.8 g

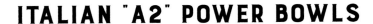

ITALIAN "A2" POWER BOWLS

Due to a genetic mutation, cow's milk cheeses contain a version of the protein casein called "A1" casein, which can be turned into an opioid (β-casomorphin-7) in our guts and cause digestive issues such as constipation, bloating, and inflammation. But the good news is that this mutation only occurs in domesticated cattle. Goat, sheep, and buffalo cheeses, or "A2" cheeses, aren't likely to cause these problems. So enjoy this summery, satisfying power bowl: it's full of antioxidant-rich veggies, magnesium-loaded pumpkin seeds, and creamy "A2" buffalo mozzarella, all dressed up in a simple pesto sauce.

CHICKEN

1 medium (200 g/7 oz) chicken breast, skinless and boneless

Salt and black pepper, to taste

1 tablespoon (15 ml) extra-virgin avocado oil or ghee

ZUCCHINI NOODLES

1 tablespoon (15 ml) extra-virgin avocado oil or ghee

1 medium (200 g/7 oz) zucchini, spiralized

PESTO DRESSING

3 tablespoons (45 ml) Macadamia Basil Pesto or any pesto on pages 198 to 199

2 tablespoons (30 ml) extra-virgin olive oil

TO ASSEMBLE

2 cups (60 g/2.1 oz) spinach, arugula, and/or watercress

1 ball (125 g/4.4 oz) buffalo mozzarella, sliced or torn into pieces

6 to 8 cherry tomatoes (85 g/3 oz), halved

10 green olives (50 g/1.8 oz whole, about 30 g/1.1 oz pitted)

1 tablespoon (8 g/0.3 oz) pumpkin seeds

Optional: black pepper and chile flakes, to taste

① To make the chicken: Tenderize the chicken breast with a mallet or a rolling pin. Season with a pinch each of salt and pepper. Heat a large skillet greased with the avocado oil over medium-high heat. Once hot, add the chicken and cook undisturbed for 5 to 7 minutes. Flip the chicken over and cook for 2 to 3 minutes. When done, transfer to a chopping board, let cool slightly, and slice.

② To make the zucchini noodles: Grease the pan in which you cooked the chicken with the of avocado oil and add the zucchini noodles. Cook for 1 to 3 minutes, then remove from the heat. Alternatively, you can serve the zucchini raw and simply drizzle some olive oil over them for extra antioxidant polyphenols.

③ To make the dressing: Combine the pesto and oil in a small bowl and mix well.

④ To assemble the salad: Divide the salad ingredients between two bowls. Top with the zucchini noodles, cooked chicken, and dressing. Finish with black pepper and chile flakes, if using. Eat immediately or refrigerate, drizzled with the dressing, for up to 1 day.

NUTRITION FACTS PER SERVING (1 BOWL):

Total carbs: 9.7 g	Fat: 59.8 g (of which saturated: 13.2 g)	SAT / MUFA / PUFA (%): 22, 68, 10
Fiber: 3.4 g	Calories: 735 kcal	Omega-6: 4.3 g
Net Carbs: 6.3 g	Macronutrient ratio: Calories from carbs (3%), protein (23%), fat (74%)	
Protein: 42.1 g		

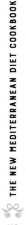

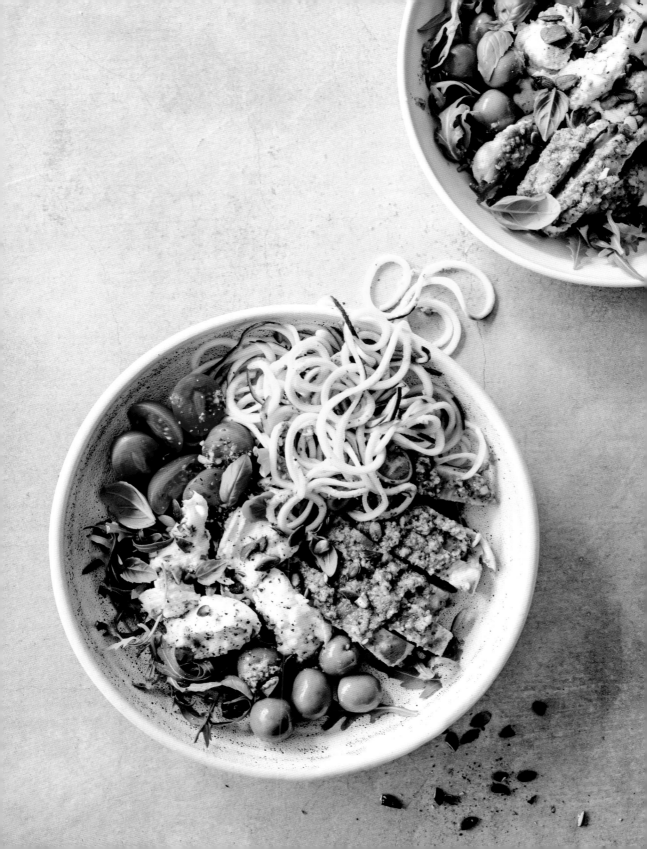

MOROCCAN POWER BOWLS

This vibrant Moroccan-inspired dish features melt-in-your-mouth lamb patties served with golden cauliflower rice and fresh spinach. Macadamia "chickpeas," coated in a harissa spice mixture and then roasted, are the cherries on the low-carb cake! What's more, this recipe's two leading ingredients, lamb and macadamia, are among the two richest sources of conjugated linoleic acid and palmitoleic acid, respectively, both of which may help reduce body fat and improve insulin sensitivity.

ROASTED HARISSA "CHICKPEAS"

1 cup (134 g/4.7 oz) macadamia nuts

2 teaspoons (10 ml) virgin coconut oil

2 teaspoons (5 g/0.2 oz) Harissa Spice Mix (page 198)

½ teaspoon paprika

Salt and black pepper, to taste

LAMB MEATBALL PATTIES

1.1 pounds (500 g) ground lamb (15% fat)

1 tablespoon (8 g/0.3 oz) Harissa Spice Mix (page 198)

2 tablespoons (14 g/0.5 oz) flax meal

1 teaspoon paprika

1 large egg

2 teaspoons (10 ml) apple cider vinegar or fresh lemon juice

1 clove garlic, minced

2 tablespoons (6 g/0.3 oz) chopped fresh mint

Salt and black pepper, to taste

1 tablespoon (15 ml) extra-virgin avocado oil or ghee

TURMERIC CAULI-RICE

1 small (500 g/1.1 lb) cauliflower

2 tablespoons (30 ml) extra-virgin avocado oil or ghee

1 teaspoon ground turmeric

½ teaspoon ground cumin

¼ teaspoon ground black pepper

Salt, to taste

TO ASSEMBLE

2 cups (60 g/2.1 oz) fresh spinach

4 teaspoons (20 ml) extra-virgin olive oil

Optional: ¼ cup (60 g/2.1 oz) goat's or sheep's milk yogurt, to serve

① Preheat the oven to 300°F (150°C) fan assisted or 340°F (170°C) conventional. Line a baking tray with parchment paper.

② To make the chickpeas: In a bowl, toss the macadamias with the coconut oil, then add the harissa spice mix, paprika, salt, and pepper. Mix well. Spread on the lined baking tray and bake for 10 to 15 minutes. Remove from the oven and set aside to cool.

③ To make the meatball patties: Place all of the ingredients, apart from the avocado oil, in a bowl. Mix to combine. Using your hands, form 16 small meatballs (about 36 g/1.3 oz each) and flatten gently into patty shapes. Place in a hot pan greased with the avocado oil and cook the patties in batches for 4 to 5 minutes per side. Transfer to a plate and set aside.

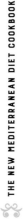

NUTRITION FACTS PER SERVING (1 BOWL):

Total carbs: 15 g	Fat: 72.1 g (of which saturated: 20.8 g)	SAT / MUFA / PUFA (%): 29, 64
Fiber: 7.7 g	Calories: 801 kcal	Omega-6/3 ratio: 2.2
Net Carbs: 7.3 g	Macronutrient ratio: Calories from carbs (4%), protein (15%), fat (81%)	
Protein: 29.9 g		

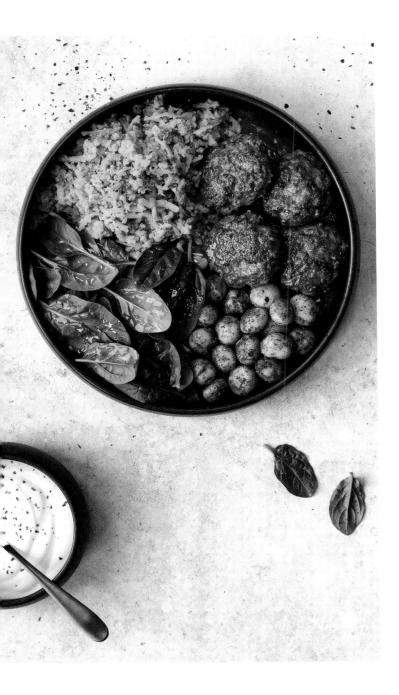

④ To make the cauli-rice: Place the florets in a food processor and process using a grating blade or the S blade until it resembles rice. Grease the same pan in which you cooked the patties with the avocado oil. Stir in the turmeric and cumin, then add the cauliflower rice and mix well. Season with salt and pepper, cook for 5 to 7 minutes, and then remove from the heat.

⑤ To assemble each serving: Place 4 patties in a bowl and add about ¾ cup (100 g/3.5 oz) of the prepared cauli-rice, ½ cup (15 g/0.5 oz) of the spinach, and ¼ cup (35 g/1.2 oz) of the macadamia "chickpeas." Drizzle each serving with 1 teaspoon of the olive oil and serve immediately with yogurt, if using. The nuts can be stored at room temperature for up to 1 week; the patties and cauli-rice can be stored in the fridge for up to 4 days. The cooked patties can also be frozen for up to 3 months.

CARB-LESS CRAB CAKES

(CONTRIBUTOR: DR. VYVYANE LOH)

This ultra-low-carb recipe was contributed by Dr. Vyvyane Loh, a board-certified obesity medicine doc and the founder of the Transform Alliance for Health, a center for metabolic medicine. Dr. Loh designed this recipe to support a patient who, she says, "wanted an easy seafood recipe to prepare in advance for a no-fuss workday lunch." These simple crab cakes definitely fit the bill! Dr. Loh also published the first-ever medical case report to examine how a Mediterranean-ketogenic diet improves cardiovascular risk markers.

CRAB CAKES

8 ounces (227 g) white crabmeat

1 large egg

2 tablespoons (16 g/0.6 oz) coconut flour

2 tablespoons (30 ml) Blender Mayonnaise (page 199) or avocado oil mayonnaise

½ teaspoon Dijon mustard

1 tablespoon (4 g/0.2 oz) chopped fresh parsley

¼ teaspoon chile flakes

Salt and black pepper, to taste

1 tablespoon (15 ml) extra-virgin avocado oil or ghee

TO SERVE

1 cup (30 g/1.1 oz) watercress, spinach, or arugula

½ cup (30 g/1.1 oz) shaved fennel (fronds reserved for garnish)

1 tablespoon (15 ml) extra-virgin olive oil

1 teaspoon fresh lemon juice

Salt and black pepper, to taste

¼ cup (35 g/1.2 oz) crushed macadamia nuts

¼ cup (34 ml) aioli made with Blender Mayonnaise (page 199), or avocado oil mayonnaise mixed with ½ clove crushed garlic

① To make the crab cakes: Place all the ingredients except the avocado oil in a mixing bowl and combine. Use a ¼-cup (60 ml) measuring cup (about 55 g/1.9 oz) to measure out each patty. The mixture will be wet, so you'll need to use your hands to form the patties. Place a large pan greased with the avocado oil over medium heat. Once hot, add as many patties as you can fit in a single layer. Cook them for 4 to 5 minutes per side, using a spatula to flip them over when they are easy to release. Repeat until all 6 patties are cooked. Set the cooked crab cakes aside.

② To assemble: Place the watercress and shaved fennel in a bowl. Drizzle with the olive oil and lemon juice and season with salt and pepper to taste. Top with the crushed macadamias. Serve with the crab cakes, using the aioli as a dip. To store, refrigerate the cooked crab cakes and salad separately for up to 3 days.

TIP: Like Dr. Loh, you can use macadamia oil to make your mayo or aioli, decreasing omega-6 to 2.5 grams.

NUTRITION FACTS PER SERVING (3 PATTIES • 2 TABLESPOONS [30 ML] AIOLI • 1 CUP [57 G/2 OZ] SIDE SALAD):

Total carbs: 7.4 g	Fat: 70 g (of which saturated: 11 g)	SAT / MUFA / PUFA (%): 16, 72, 12
Fiber: 3.8 g	Calories: 764 kcal	Omega-6: 6.0 g
Net Carbs: 3.6 g	Macronutrient ratio: Calories from carbs (2%), protein (15%), fat (83%)	
Protein: 28.7 g		

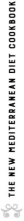

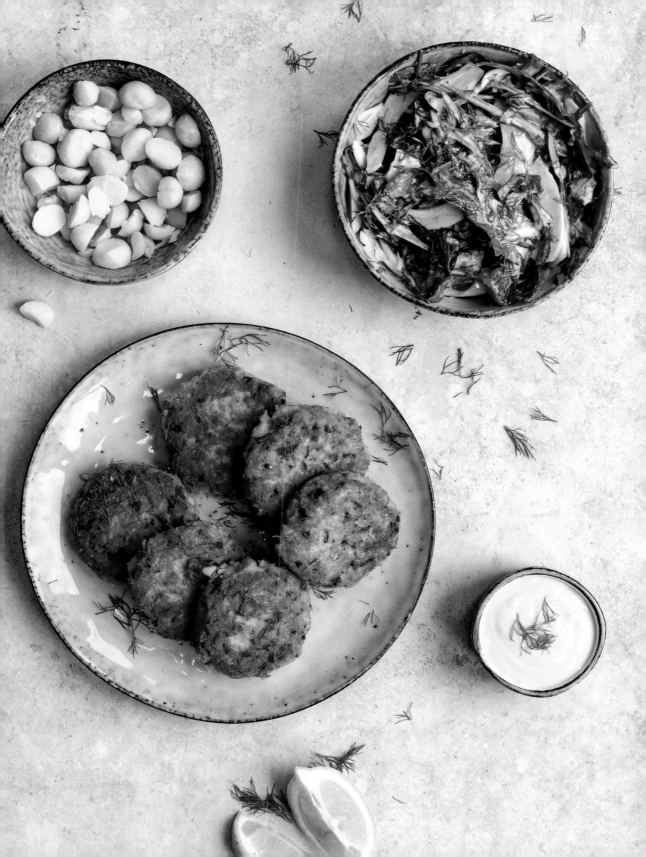

THYROID-FRIENDLY SALMON FISH CAKES WITH FENNEL "NOODLES" AND BRAZIL NUT PESTO

(CONTRIBUTOR: MARTINA SLAJEROVA)

Packed with healthy fats and thyroid-supporting micronutrients, this tasty lunch box option is optimized to boost your metabolic health. Salmon cakes, fragrant fennel "noodles," and Brazil Nut Watercress Pesto (page 199) together provide loads of selenium, magnesium, and other thyroid-supporting micronutrients.

SALMON PATTIES

12 ounces (340 g) canned drained salmon

2 large eggs

1½ tablespoons (12 g/0.4 oz) coconut flour

1 tablespoon (7 g/0.3 oz) flax meal

2 tablespoons (8 g/0.3 oz) chopped fresh parsley

1 tablespoon (4 g/0.2 oz) chopped fresh dill

1 tablespoon (15 ml) fresh lemon juice

1 teaspoon lemon zest

1 clove garlic, minced

2 medium (30 g/1.1 oz) spring onions

Pinch of salt and black pepper

1 tablespoon (15 ml) extra-virgin avocado oil or ghee

FENNEL "NOODLES"

1 large or 2 small (400 g/14.1 oz) fennel bulbs

1 tablespoon (15 ml) extra-virgin avocado oil or ghee

Salt and black pepper, to taste

½ cup (120 ml) Brazil Nut Watercress Pesto (page 199)

① To make the patties: Place all the ingredients except the avocado oil in a mixing bowl and combine. Use a ¼-cup (60 ml) measuring cup (about 58 g/2 oz) to create 9 patties.

② Heat a pan greased with the avocado oil over medium heat. Once hot, add as many patties as you can fit in a single layer. Cook for 4 to 5 minutes per side, using a spatula to flip them over once they are easy to release. Set the patties aside.

③ To make the fennel noodles: Slice the fennel into thin "noodles," or use the slicing blade in your food processor. Grease a skillet with the avocado oil and add the fennel noodles. Cook over medium-high heat for 2 to 3 minutes and add salt and pepper to taste, then set aside. Transfer to a mixing bowl and combine with about half (¼ cup/60 ml) of the pesto.

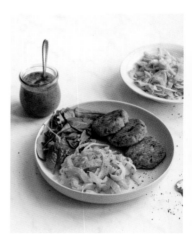

④ Serve the noodles with the patties and use the remaining pesto for dipping. To store, refrigerate the cooked patties and fennel noodles separately for up to 4 days. The patties can be frozen for up to 3 months.

NUTRITION FACTS PER SERVING (3 PATTIES • FENNEL NOODLES • PESTO):

Total carbs: 15.7 g	Fat: 43.8 g (of which saturated: 8.1 g)	SAT / MUFA / PUFA (%): 18, 65, 17
Fiber: 7.1 g	Calories: 600 kcal	Omega-6/3 ratio: 2.0
Net Carbs: 8.6 g	Macronutrient ratio: Calories from carbs (6%), protein (27%), fat (67%)	
Protein: 40.1 g		

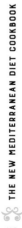

CRISPY GINGER MACKEREL LUNCH BOWLS

We make this Thai-inspired dish the Mediterranean way, with lots of omega-3 fats and low-carb veggies. Here, juicy mackerel's oily goodness is enhanced with a quick, creamy dressing made with anti-inflammatory thai-hini (sorry, we couldn't resist), ginger, and fresh citrus juices. Add a tangle of kelp noodles and strew over a handful of crushed macadamias, and you've got a warming lunch for two that's ready in a bare 15 minutes.

GINGER THAI-HINI DRESSING

1 tablespoon (6 g/0.2 oz) grated fresh ginger

1 tablespoon (15 ml) fresh lime or lemon juice

2 tablespoons (30 ml) extra-virgin olive oil

2 tablespoons (32 g/1.1 oz) tahini

1 clove garlic, minced

MACKEREL

2 mackerel fillets (250 g/8.8 oz)

Pinch of salt and black pepper

1 tablespoon (15 ml) extra-virgin avocado oil or ghee

TO ASSEMBLE

16 to 20 spears (200 g/7 oz) asparagus

1 small (100 g/3.5 oz) bok choy, halved

1 tablespoon (15 ml) extra-virgin olive oil

½ pack (170 g/6 oz) kelp noodles, drained

¼ cup (34 g/1.2 oz) macadamia nuts, roughly chopped

1 small (5 g/0.5 oz) chile pepper, sliced

1 tablespoon (4 g/0.2 oz) chopped fresh cilantro or parsley

① To make the dressing: Place the dressing ingredients in a bowl and mix to combine. If the dressing is too thick, add a dash of water.

② To make the mackerel: Cut 2 or 3 diagonal slits in the skin of the mackerel and season with salt and pepper on both sides. Heat a skillet greased with the avocado oil over medium heat. Add the mackerel fillets and cook for 2 to 3 minutes per side. Remove from the heat and set aside.

③ To assemble: Place the asparagus and the bok choy in a steamer (or a saucepan with a steamer colander inside) and fill with about 1 cup (240 ml) of water and bring to a boil. Cover with a lid and steam for 3 to 5 minutes, until crisp-tender. Remove the lid and let the steam escape.

④ Divide the steamed veggies between two bowls, drizzle with the olive oil, and season with salt and pepper. Add the prepared kelp noodles and top with the mackerel. Drizzle with the dressing and top with the macadamias, chile pepper, and cilantro. Eat warm or refrigerate for up to 1 day.

FUN FACT

This may sound like science fiction, but it's true: Scientists at Harvard engineered mutant mice that can make omega-3 fats in their bodies. They showed that having a better omega-6/3 ratio alone, with no difference in diet, caused the mice to be leaner, have healthier microbiomes, and be less prone to cancer. You can't go wrong by adding yummy omega-3-rich mackerel to your diet!

NUTRITION FACTS PER SERVING (1 BOWL):

Total carbs: 13.3 g	Fat: 66.2 g (of which saturated: 11 g)	SAT / MUFA / PUFA (%): 17, 63, 20
Fiber: 6.5 g	Calories: 751 kcal	Omega-6/3 ratio: 1.9 ☺
Net Carbs: 6.8 g	Macronutrient ratio: Calories from carbs	
Protein: 30.5 g	(4%), protein (16%), fat (80%)	

SALMON POKE BOWLS

(CONTRIBUTOR: BEATRICE PASQUIER)

This twist on a popular Hawaiian summer staple, made with cauliflower rice and soy-free coconut aminos, was contributed by Ms. Beatrice Pasquier, who lost 30 pounds (13.6 kg) and reversed her prediabetes in her first two months on a ketogenic diet. Her weight loss has continued steadily since then. She remains slim, prediabetes-free, and "dance-in-my-kitchen" happy, particularly while preparing this favorite lunch with her husband, Paul. Add crunchy cucumber, creamy avocado, and nori flakes and you've got the perfect dish for hot summer days, or dancing in your kitchen!

(Note: Consuming raw fish may increase your risk of food-borne illness. Be sure to handle it carefully, and only use fish from reputable sources.)

MARINATED SALMON

8 ounces (227 g) sushi-grade wild salmon

1 tablespoon (15 ml) coconut aminos

2 tablespoons (30 ml) extra-virgin olive oil

1 teaspoon toasted sesame oil

½ to 1 teaspoon chile flakes

1 tablespoon (9 g/0.3 oz) sesame seeds

2 medium (15 g/0.5 oz) spring onions, sliced

CAULI-RICE

½ medium (250 g/8.8 oz) cauliflower

2 tablespoons (30 ml) avocado oil or ghee

1 tablespoon (15 ml) fresh lemon juice

Salt and black pepper, to taste

TO ASSEMBLE

1 large (200 g/7 oz) avocado, cubed

1 medium (200 g/7 oz) cucumber, cubed

2 tablespoons (30 ml) extra-virgin olive oil

½ nori sheet, crumbled or cut into small pieces

① To make the salmon: Cut the salmon into small cubes. In a small bowl, combine the salmon and the remaining marinade ingredients. Mix well, then set aside while you cook the cauli-rice.

② To make the cauli-rice: Place the florets in a food processor and process using a grating blade or the S blade until it resembles rice. Grease a pan with the avocado oil and add the cauli-rice. Cook over medium-high heat for 5 to 7 minutes, stirring frequently to prevent burning. Remove from the heat. Add the fresh lemon juice, season with salt and pepper, and set aside.

③ To assemble the poke bowls: Divide the cauli-rice between two bowls, and top each with half of the marinated salmon mixture, avocado, and cucumber. Drizzle with the olive oil, sprinkle with the crumbled nori, and serve.

NUTRITION FACTS PER SERVING (1 BOWL):

Total carbs: 20.3 g	Fat: 54.0 g (of which saturated: 7.8 g)	SAT / MUFA / PUFA (%): 15, 68, 17
Fiber: 11.1 g	Calories: 668 kcal	Omega-6/3 ratio: 2.9
Net Carbs: 9.3 g	Macronutrient ratio: Calories from carbs (6%), protein (19%), fat (75%)	
Protein: 30.9 g		

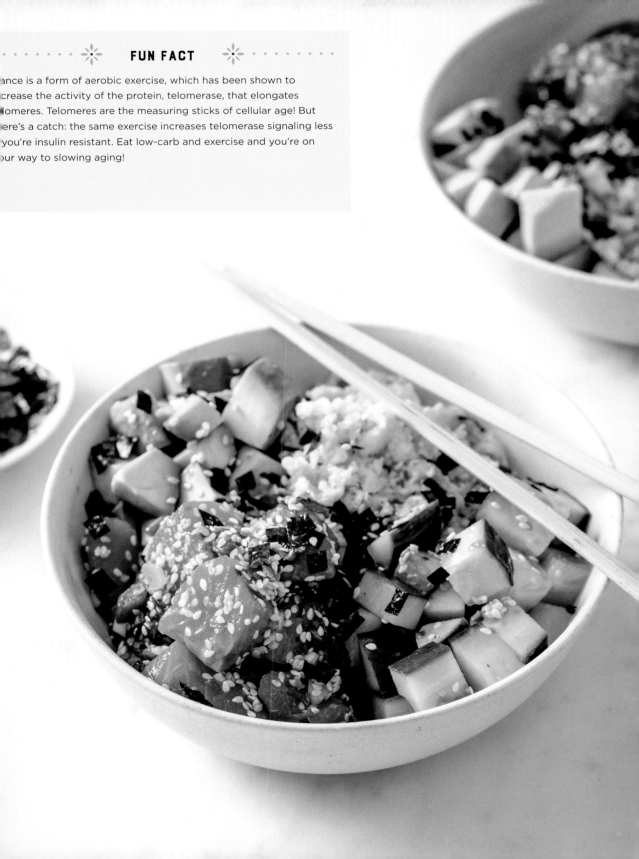

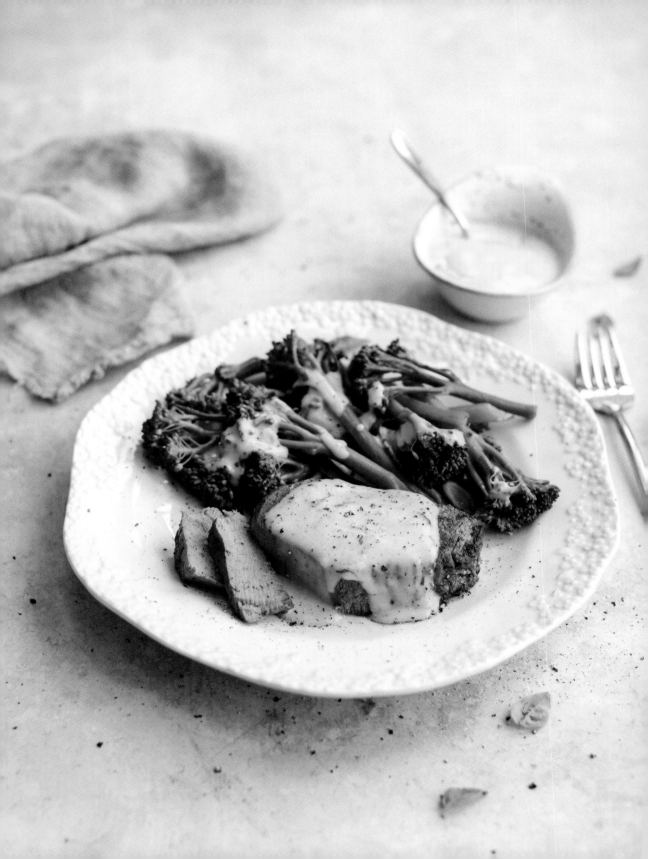

CHAPTER 6

DINNERS

◄ *Rumination-Free Steak with
Creamy Béarnaise Sauce (page 156)*

HALLOUMI CURRY SKILLET

Salty, chewy Halloumi cheese makes a delicious veggie alternative to meat in homemade curries. That said, this creamy one-pot meal works with any protein, so switch things up if you're not a vegetarian. It's also super low in inflammatory omega-6, and if you use ghee instead of avocado oil, you can drop the omega-6 to 3 percent (less than 0.5 gram)!

2 packs (500 g/1.1 lb) Halloumi cheese

2 tablespoons (30 ml) extra-virgin avocado oil or ghee

1 teaspoon onion powder

½ teaspoon garlic powder

1½ tablespoons (10 g/0.4 oz) mild or medium curry powder

½ teaspoon ground turmeric

¼ teaspoon ground black pepper

¼ cup (60 g/2.1 oz) tomato paste

½ cup (120 ml) coconut milk

1 cup (240 ml) water

1 small (450 g/1 lb) cauliflower, cut into small florets

Salt, to taste

2 tablespoons (16 g/0.6 oz) coconut flour

Fresh cilantro or parsley, to serve

Optional: cauli-rice (page 166), shirataki rice, or Quick Low-Carb Bread (page 38)

① Cut the Halloumi into 8 slices, each about ¾ inch (2 cm) thick. Heat a large skillet greased with the avocado oil over medium-high heat. Cook the Halloumi slices in batches, turning them so they cook on all sides. At first, they will be hard to turn, but once they develop a crispy golden crust, it's time to turn them and it will be easy to do so. When done, transfer to a plate and keep warm.

② To the skillet in which you browned the Halloumi, add the onion powder, garlic powder, curry powder, turmeric, pepper, tomato paste, coconut milk, and water. Bring to a boil and add the cauliflower. Cover with a lid and cook until fork-tender, 7 to 10 minutes. Season with salt to taste.

③ Remove the lid and mix in the coconut flour to thicken the sauce. Finally, add the browned Halloumi and cook briefly to heat through. Serve warm on its own, or with cauli-rice or some Quick Keto Bread. Store in the fridge for up to 5 days.

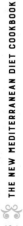
NUTRITION FACTS PER SERVING:

Total carbs: 13.8 g	Fat: 48.1 g (of which saturated: 28.2 g)	SAT / MUFA / PUFA (%): 59, 36, 5
Fiber: 4.8 g	Calories: 590 kcal	Omega-6: 1.3 g
Net Carbs: 8.8 g	Macronutrient ratio: Calories from carbs (6%), protein (20%), fat (74%)	
Protein: 29.2 g		

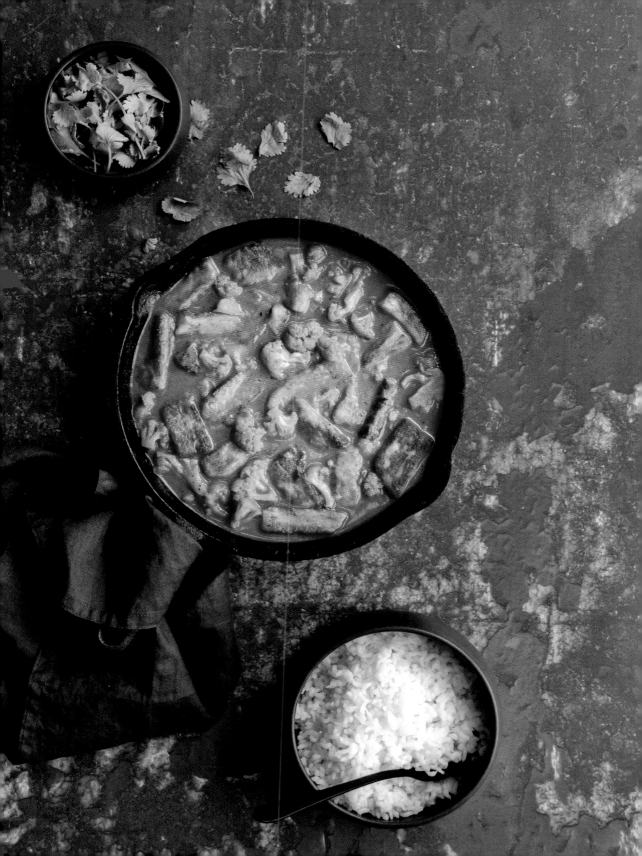

EGGPLANT MANICOTTI

This Italian-American dish will show you it's easier to make keto pasta substitutes than you think! It features eggplant slices stuffed with a delicious herbed-cheese filling baked in a homemade marinara sauce and topped with even more gooey, melty cheese. Don't feel guilty about enjoying it, either: a ten-week placebo-controlled human study found that Pecorino Romano, which is naturally rich in the fatty acid conjugated linoleic acid, reduced markers of inflammation and cardiovascular risk.

2 medium (600 g/1.3 lb) eggplants

2 tablespoons (30 ml) extra-virgin avocado oil or ghee, divided

Pinch of salt and black pepper

1 pack (250 g/8.8 oz) soft goat's or sheep's cheese

1 large egg

Pinch of ground nutmeg

7 ounces (200 g) frozen spinach, thawed and squeezed dry (weight excludes water squeezed out)

1 clove garlic, crushed

2 tablespoons (8 g/0.3 oz) chopped fresh basil

2 tablespoons (8 g/0.3 oz) chopped fresh parsley

½ cup (40 g/1.4 oz) grated Pecorino Romano or other Italian-style hard cheese made from sheep's or goat's milk, divided

1 cup (113 g/4 oz) grated buffalo mozzarella cheese, divided

¼ cup (60 ml) Blender Marinara Sauce (page 198)

① Preheat the oven to 400°F (200°C) fan assisted or 425°F (220°C) conventional. Line a two baking trays with parchment paper.

② Cut the eggplants into about ½-inch (1 cm)-thick slices; you should have a total of 12 slices. Place the slices on the baking trays. Brush with half of the avocado oil, and season with salt and pepper. Bake for 20 to 25 minutes, rotating the tray halfway through to ensure even cooking. Remove from the oven and let them cool down. Reduce the temperature to 355°F (180°C) fan assisted or 400°F (200°C) conventional.

③ Meanwhile, combine the soft cheese, egg, nutmeg, spinach, garlic, basil, and parsley in a large bowl. Add half of the Pecorino and half of the mozzarella. Mix well.

④ Grease a baking dish with the remaining 1 tablespoon (15 ml) avocado oil. Place 2 heaping tablespoons of the filling (about 50 g/1.8 oz) onto each eggplant slice and roll up. Repeat until all of the slices and filling are used. Place the eggplant rolls in the greased baking dish, seam-side down. Spread the marinara sauce on top of the rolls and sprinkle with the remaining Pecorino Romano and remaining mozzarella.

⑤ Bake for 20 to 25 minutes, until the eggplant is cooked and the cheese has melted. Eat warm. To store, refrigerate for up to 5 days.

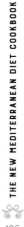

NUTRITION FACTS PER SERVING:

Total carbs: 14.3 g	Fat: 32.6 g (of which saturated: 15.6 g)	SAT / MUFA / PUFA (%): 48, 44, 8
Fiber: 6.3 g	Calories: 447 kcal	Omega-6: 1.75 g
Net Carbs: 8 g	Macronutrient ratio: Calories from carbs (7%), protein (25%), fat (68%)	
Protein: 27.1 g		

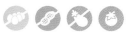

TRICOLORE PASTA BOWL

This is a great go-to meal for busy days. In just 10 minutes you'll have a big bowl of antioxidants and healthy fats in front of you. This beautiful green (zucchini, basil), red (marinara sauce), and white (mozzarella) dish symbolizes the flag of Italy, also called the *il Tricolore*. Plus, buffalo milk has 50 percent more healthy fat than cow's milk, and a greater antioxidant capacity, too, which is why we use buffalo mozzarella.

1 tablespoon (15 ml) extra-virgin avocado oil

2 medium (400 g/14.1 oz) zucchini, spiralized

¼ cup (60 ml) extra-virgin olive oil

¼ cup (60 ml) Blender Marinara Sauce (page 198)

3.5 ounces (100 g) buffalo mozzarella, sliced

10 pitted Kalamata or green olives (30 g/1.1 oz)

Fresh basil leaves, salt, and pepper, to taste

Optional: Pecorino Romano flakes, to serve

① Grease a skillet with the avocado oil. Once hot, add the zucchini noodles. Cook for 1 to 3 minutes, until desired doneness. (You can even skip this step and simply serve them uncooked.) Mix the "zoodles" with the olive oil, followed by all of the remaining ingredients. Sprinkle over the Pecorino Romano flakes, if using. Serve immediately or store in the fridge for up to 1 day.

TIPS: For extra protein, add more mozzarella or diced cooked chicken. ❖ For extra fats, add some diced avocado or pesto. ❖ Or use pesto in place of the marinara sauce; this will also make this meal nightshade-free.

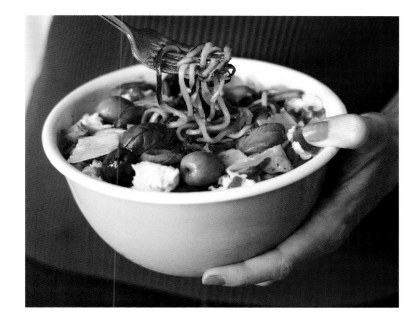

NUTRITION FACTS PER SERVING:

Total carbs: 9.9 g	Fat: 50.6 g (of which saturated: 11 g)	SAT / MUFA / PUFA (%): 22, 68, 10
Fiber: 2.9 g	Calories: 542 kcal	Omega-6: 4.6 g
Net Carbs: 7 g	Macronutrient ratio: Calories from carbs (5%), protein (11%), fat (84%)	
Protein: 15.1 g		

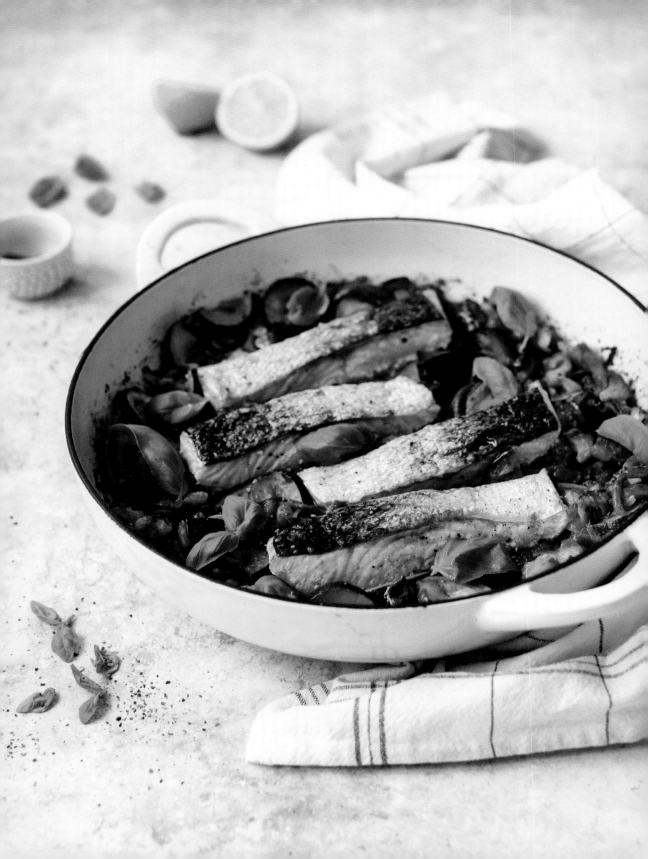

SALMON RATATOUILLE SKILLET

One-pot meals make excellent weekday dinner solutions: they let you enjoy a wider range of nutritious foods with way less work—and way less cleanup afterward. And you really can't mess them up: Just toss everything in one pot and cook. This recipe takes its inspiration from the vegetarian French casserole, *ratatouille,* which is big on low-carb vegetables such as eggplant, green pepper, and zucchini, but we've turned it into a complete meal by adding wild salmon for healthy fats and protein.

2 tablespoons (30 ml) extra-virgin avocado oil

1 small (70 g/2.5 oz) red onion, sliced

2 cloves garlic, minced

1 medium (120 g/4.2 oz) green bell pepper, sliced

1 medium (300 g/10.6 oz) eggplant, cut into ½-inch (1 cm) pieces

1 cup (240 g/8.5 oz) canned tomatoes

¼ cup (60 ml) water

2 tablespoons (30 ml) fresh lemon juice, divided

1 medium (200 g/7 oz) zucchini, cut into ½-inch (1 cm) pieces

1 teaspoon dried Italian herbs

Salt and black pepper, to taste

4 small fillets (500 g/1.1 lb) wild salmon, skin on (125 g/4.4 oz each)

¼ cup (60 ml) extra-virgin olive oil

Chopped or whole-leaf fresh basil, to taste

① Heat an ovenproof skillet (with a lid) greased with the avocado oil over medium heat. Add the onion and cook for 5 minutes. Add the garlic, bell pepper, eggplant, tomatoes, water, and 1 tablespoon (15 ml) of the fresh lemon juice.

② Bring to a boil, and then reduce the heat to low. Cover with a lid and cook for about 8 minutes to reduce the sauce. Add the zucchini, Italian herbs, salt, and pepper. Stir to combine, cover again, and cook for about 5 minutes.

③ Preheat the oven to 400°F (200°C) fan assisted or 425°F (220°C) conventional. Add the salmon fillets, skin-side up, to the pot and drizzle with the remaining 1 tablespoon (15 ml) lemon juice. Place in the oven and cook for about 10 minutes, until the salmon is cooked through. For crispier skin, broil on high for the last 2 to 3 minutes.

④ To serve, drizzle everything with the olive oil and sprinkle with the basil. This is best eaten within a day, but it can be stored in the fridge for up to 3 days.

NUTRITION FACTS PER SERVING:

Total carbs: 11.8 g	Fat: 28.5 g (of which saturated: 4.4 g)	SAT / MUFA / PUFA (%): 15, 71, 14
Fiber: 4.8 g	Calories: 417 kcal	Omega-6/3 ratio: 0.7 ☺
Net Carbs: 7 g	Macronutrient ratio: Calories from carbs (7%), protein (29%), fat (64%)	
Protein: 29.5 g		

SHRIMP SCAMPI

There are two secrets hidden in this healthy twist on the classic Italian recipe for shrimp scampi. The first secret is this: To make perfect low-carb pasta, use shirataki noodles and cook them in the buttery, lemony sauce for a few minutes so they really soak up all the flavors. And second, this dish has three sources of "odd-chain" saturated fats that act like anti-inflammatory omega-3 fats. Research suggests that these nutritionally rare "odd-chain" saturated fatty acids are concentrated in shrimp, ghee, and cheeses such as Pecorino Romano, and can activate fat-burning PPAR proteins, protect mitochondria, and reduce inflammation.

¼ cup (57 g/2 oz) ghee

¼ cup (60 ml) extra-virgin avocado oil

4 cloves garlic, minced

¼ cup (60 ml) fresh lemon juice

Salt and black pepper, to taste

½ teaspoon dried oregano or ½ tablespoon chopped fresh oregano

1.3 pounds (600 g) raw, peeled and deveined shrimp

4 packs (400 g/14.1 oz) shirataki noodles or shirataki fettucine

2 large (500 g/1.1 lb) zucchini, spiralized

1 cup (80 g/2.8 oz) grated Pecorino Romano

¼ cup (15 g/0.5 oz) chopped fresh parsley

① Place the ghee and avocado oil in a large skillet or a shallow casserole dish suitable for stovetop use. Add the garlic and cook over medium-high heat for about 1 minute. Add the lemon juice, a pinch each of salt and pepper, and the oregano. Bring to a boil. Add the shrimp and cook for 2 to 3 minutes, until pink and opaque. Do not overcook. Use a slotted spoon to transfer the cooked shrimp to a plate and set aside.

② Add the shirataki noodles to the skillet and cook for 3 to 5 minutes. Add the zucchini noodles and cook for 1 to 2 minutes (or until desired doneness). Remove from the heat and add the grated Pecorino and fresh parsley. Toss to combine and season to taste if needed.

③ Add the shrimp back to the pot. Optionally, place the casserole dish under a broiler for 1 to 2 minutes to melt the cheese. Divide among four serving bowls and eat warm. Store in the fridge for up to 3 days.

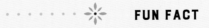

FUN FACT

Linus Pauling, the only person to ever win *two* independent Nobel Prizes, believed vitamin C is essential for heart health. It's therefore not surprising that goats, an animal that makes 150 times the human RDA of vitamin C within their own bodies, don't tend to get heart disease. Keeping your carbs low helps you absorb more vitamin C.

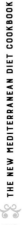

NUTRITION FACTS PER SERVING:

Total carbs: 10.3 g	Fat: 36.1 g (of which saturated: 14.6 g)	SAT / MUFA / PUFA (%): 40, 49, 11
Fiber: 3 g	Calories: 472 kcal	Omega-6/3 ratio: 2.5
Net Carbs: 7.3 g	Macronutrient ratio: Calories from carbs (6%), protein (26%), fat (68%)	
Protein: 30.6 g		

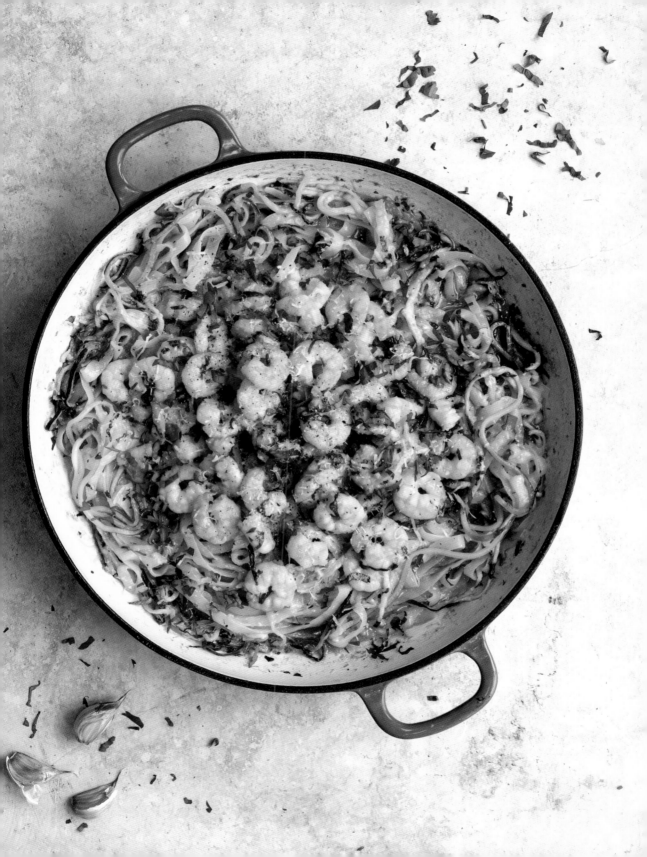

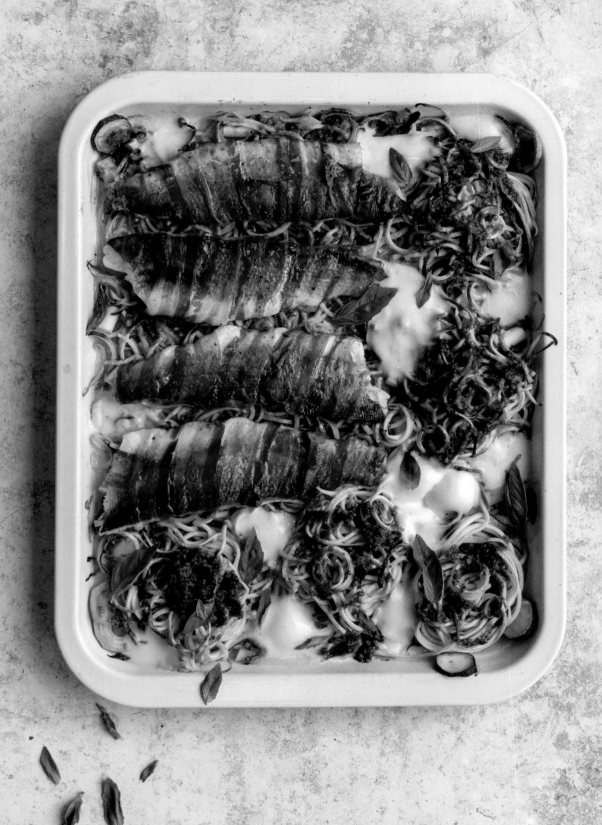

PANCETTA-WRAPPED SEA BASS SHEET PAN

(CONTRIBUTOR: IVOR CUMMINS)

This one-pan meal, featuring tender sea bass wrapped in crispy pancetta and baked with pesto-zucchini nests plus creamy mozzarella, was contributed by Ivor Cummins, also known as the "Fat Emperor." A biomedical engineer by training, Ivor dedicated himself to studying nutrition science when he was diagnosed with fatty liver disease. He quickly reversed his condition and has since become a pioneer in nutrition science. With less than 5 percent carbs, this dish is an elegant, heart-healthy take on surf and turf!

4 medium (800 g/1.76 lb) zucchini and/or yellow summer squash, spiralized

6 ounces (170 g) buffalo mozzarella, cubed or torn

¼ cup (60 ml) Macadamia Basil Pesto or any pesto on pages 198 to 199

¼ cup (60 ml) extra-virgin avocado oil

12 slices (140 g/5 oz) pancetta or thinly sliced bacon

4 fillets (340 g/12 oz) sea bass or sea bream

Salt and black pepper, to taste

Chopped fresh herbs such as basil, oregano, and/or thyme, for garnish

① Preheat the oven to 400°F (200°C) fan assisted or 425°F (220°C) conventional.

② Using the zucchini noodles, create several nests by wrapping the noodles around your index and middle fingers. Place the nests on a baking tray and top with the mozzarella pieces and add any leftover noodles that were too short to create nests with.

③ In a small bowl, mix the pesto and the avocado oil. Drizzle the "zoodles" with the pesto-oil mixture. Wrap 3 pancetta slices around each of the sea bass fillets and place in the baking tray next to the nests. Season with salt and pepper and bake for 7 to 10 minutes, until the fish is cooked through and the pancetta is crispy.

④ Eat warm garnished with the fresh herbs. Store in the fridge for up to 3 days.

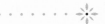 **FUN FACT**

Vasa vasorum are the blood vessels that that wrap around your coronary arteries, like the pancetta wraps around this sea bass. When the inside of your blood vessels get damaged by inflammation, the vasa vasorum grow inward and can deposit plaque-building substances into your artery walls. This is the outside-in model of cardiovascular disease.

NUTRITION FACTS PER SERVING:

Total carbs: 8.3 g	Fat: 44.3 g (of which saturated: 11.3 g)	SAT / MUFA / PUFA (%): 26, 60, 14
Fiber: 2.3 g	Calories: 568 kcal	Omega-6/3 ratio: 3.0
Net Carbs: 6 g	Macronutrient ratio: Calories from carbs (4%), protein (25%), fat (71%)	
Protein: 35.5 g		

SPICY COD & VEG SHEET PAN

This quick and easy Asian-style fish tray bake is infused with garlic, ginger, lime juice, and a kick of chile peppers. Add more chile if you like it spicy. We promise, the dish will be just as anti-inflammatory.

ASIAN MARINADE

3 tablespoons (45 ml) fresh lime or lemon juice

½ cup (120 ml) extra-virgin avocado oil

1 teaspoon toasted sesame oil

2 cloves garlic, crushed

1 tablespoon (15 ml) coconut aminos

1 tablespoon (6 g/0.2 oz) grated fresh ginger or ¼ teaspoon ground ginger

½ teaspoon salt, or to taste

¼ teaspoon black pepper, or to taste

TRAY BAKE

4 fillets (600 g/1.3 lb) cod or any white fish

1.3 pounds (600 g) broccoli, cut into small florets and halved, or broccolini

1 small (14 g/0.5 oz) red chile pepper, sliced

Optional: fresh cilantro or parsley, to serve

① To make the marinade: Combine all of the marinade ingredients in a small bowl.

② To make the tray bake: Place the fish fillets in a bowl. Pour half of the marinade over the fillets and refrigerate for at least 30 minutes or overnight. Reserve the other half of the marinade.

③ When ready to bake, preheat the oven to 350°F (175°C) fan assisted or 380°F (195°C) conventional.

④ Broccoli burns easily; make sure to slice the florets to help them cook evenly without burning. Place the broccoli on a baking tray and drizzle with the reserved marinade. Bake for 10 to 12 minutes.

⑤ Increase the temperature to 400°F (200°C) fan assisted or 425°F (220°C) conventional. Add the fish, including any marinade left in the bowl, and sliced chile pepper, then bake for 7 to 10 minutes (the exact time depends on the thickness of the fillets).

⑥ Eat warm with a sprinkling of fresh herbs, if using, or let cool and store in the fridge for up to 3 days.

FUN FACT

While there are multiple ideas as to how we evolved big brains, one of the most compelling is that the evolution of the large human brain depended on a rich source of DHA from the land/water interface. Our brains grew when our ancestors migrated from the African inland to the African coast. Basically, seafood made us nerds!

NUTRITION FACTS PER SERVING (1 FILLET • VEGETABLES):

Total carbs: 12.1 g	Fat: 30 g (of which saturated: 3.6 g)	SAT / MUFA / PUFA (%): 12, 70, 18
Fiber: 4.1 g	Calories: 433 kcal	Omega-6/3 ratio: 6.0
Net Carbs: 8 g	Macronutrient ratio: Calories from carbs (8%), protein (29%), fat (63%)	
Protein: 31.2 g		

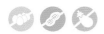
CRISPY SALMON PICCATA

We think salmon skin is the best part of the fish! This recipe shows you how to make the perfect salmon fillet—panfried until tender, but with a crispy, oily skin that knocks the flavor socks off any potato chip, and served in a lemony, caper-studded cream sauce. For a complete meal, serve it with steamed asparagus, zucchini noodles, broccoli, green beans, or cooked leafy greens.

4 medium fillets (600 g/1.3 lb) wild salmon (150 g/5.3 oz each), skin on

3 tablespoons (45 ml) extra-virgin avocado oil or ghee, divided

Salt and black pepper, to taste

2 cloves garlic, minced

1 tablespoon (15 ml) apple cider vinegar or brine from capers

¼ cup (60 ml) fresh lemon juice (for a milder flavor, you can substitute 2 tablespoons/30 ml with water or chicken stock)

½ cup (120 ml) goat's cream or heavy whipping cream

¼ cup (35 g/1.2 oz) capers, drained

2 tablespoons (8 g/0.3 oz) chopped fresh parsley and/or dill

Lemon slices, for garnish

Optional: grilled or steamed asparagus or broccoli, to serve

① Using a sharp knife, carefully remove the skins from the salmon. Place the skins in a hot skillet greased with 1 tablespoon (15 ml) of the avocado oil. Season with a pinch of salt. Cook over medium-high heat until the skins are crispy, 3 to 5 minutes. Remove from the pan and set aside.

② Season the salmon fillets with a pinch of salt and pepper. Grease the same skillet with 1 tablespoon (15 ml) of the avocado oil. Add the salmon and cook over medium heat for 3 to 4 minutes per side, until browned and cooked through. Remove from the pan and set aside.

③ Grease the skillet again with the remaining 1 tablespoon (15 ml) oil, add the garlic, and cook for 1 minute. Add the vinegar, lemon juice, and cream. Bring to a boil. Cook for 1 minute, then add the capers and parsley (you can reserve some for garnish). Return the salmon fillets to the skillet and cook briefly to heat through.

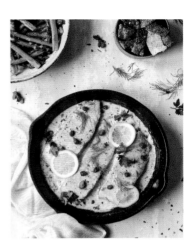

④ Add the lemon slices and serve with the crispy salmon skins and low-carb veggies, if using. The is best eaten within a day, but it can be stored in the fridge for up to 3 days.

NUTRITION FACTS PER SERVING:

Total carbs: 3 g	Fat: 31.5 g (of which saturated: 10 g)	SAT / MUFA / PUFA (%): 32, 53, 15
Fiber: 0.5 g	Calories: 425 kcal	Omega-6/3 ratio: 0.4 ☺
Net Carbs: 2.5 g	Macronutrient ratio: Calories from carbs (2%), protein (29%), fat (69%)	
Protein: 30.8 g		

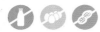
COCONUT SHRIMP SKILLET

Craving those sweet-and-crispy coconut-battered shrimp that are off-limits on a keto diet? Don't worry, you'll be able to get your fix with this seven-ingredient, one-pan, low-carb skillet meal! If you've never had melted coconut butter with shrimp before, you're in for a surprising treat: the subtle sweetness of both the coconut butter and the shrimp amplify and complement each other. This is best served over zucchini noodles. (Nutrition note: A singular "zucchina" contains as much potassium as a banana!)

2 tablespoons (30 ml) extra-virgin avocado oil or ghee, divided

2 medium (30 g/1.1 oz) spring onions, white and green parts separated, chopped

3 cloves garlic, minced

1 medium (14 g/0.5 oz) red chile pepper, seeds removed and finely chopped

8.8 ounces (250 g) raw peeled shrimp

¼ cup (64 g/2.2 oz) coconut butter (coconut manna)

Salt and black pepper, to taste

2 tablespoons (30 ml) extra-virgin olive oil

2 medium (400 g/14.1 oz) zucchini, spiralized

① Heat a skillet greased with 1 tablespoon (15 ml) of the avocado oil over medium-high heat. Add the white parts of the spring onions, garlic, and chile pepper. Cook for 1 to 2 minutes, until fragrant. Add the shrimp and cook for about 2 minutes, until opaque (do not overcook). Add the coconut butter, stir to combine, and season with salt and pepper. Remove from the heat and set aside.

② Use a spatula to transfer the entire contents of the pan to a bowl. Drizzle with the olive oil and season to taste. Sprinkle with the reserved spring onions.

③ Grease the pan in which you cooked the shrimp with the remaining 1 tablespoon (15 ml) avocado oil. Add the "zoodles" and cook for 1 to 3 minutes, tossing to ensure even cooking. Top with the cooked shrimp, then remove from the heat.

④ Serve warm or let cool and store in the fridge in a sealed container for up to 3 days.

NUTRITION FACTS PER SERVING:

Total carbs: 16.8 g	Fat: 46.8 g (of which saturated: 19.5 g)	SAT / MUFA / PUFA (%): 42, 49, 9
Fiber: 7.4 g	Calories: 555 kcal	Omega-6/3 ratio: 3.4
Net Carbs: 9.4 g	Macronutrient ratio: Calories from carbs (7%), protein (17%), fat (76%)	
Protein: 23.1 g		

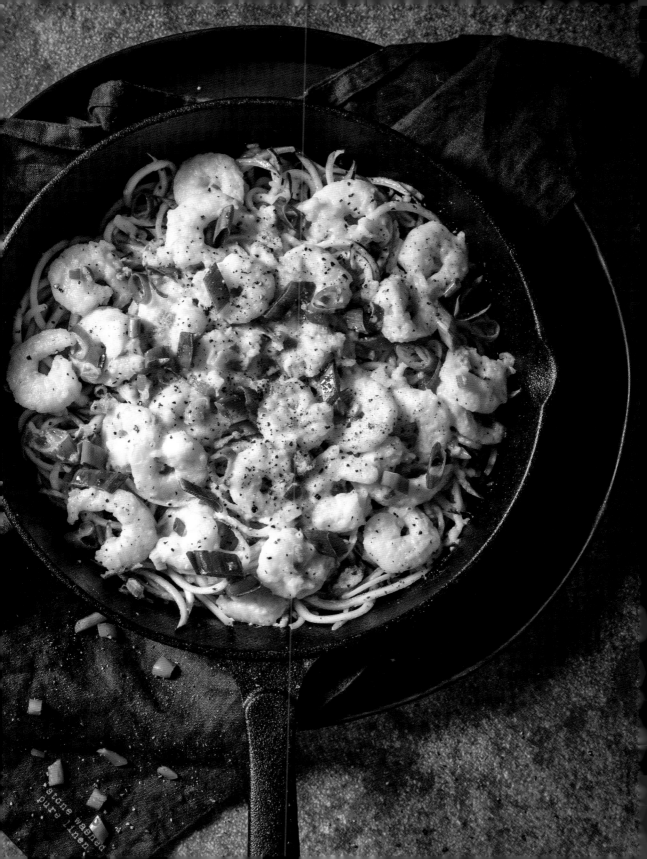

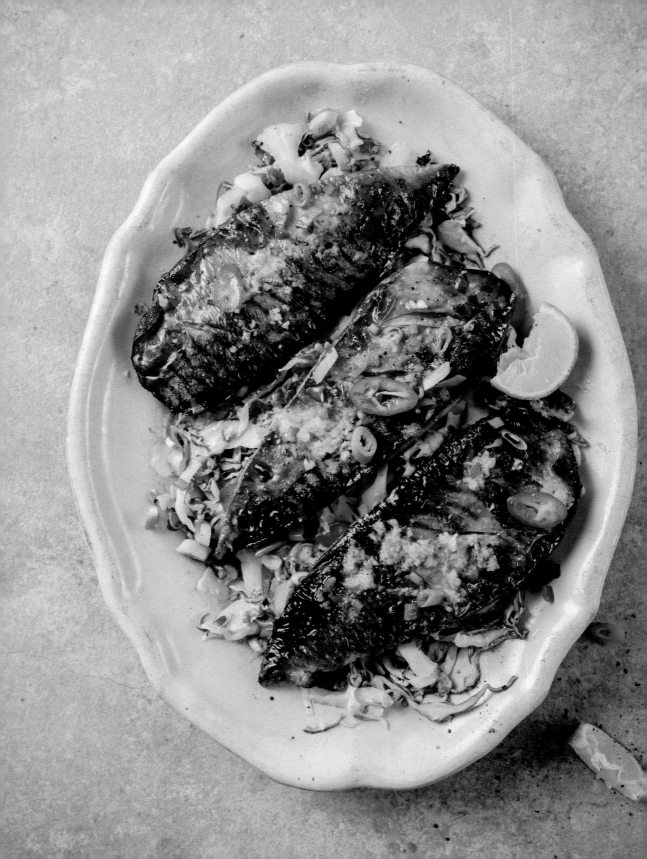

CHILE-LIME MACKEREL WITH CILANTRO SLAW

Mackerel is a delicious oily fish with an intense flavor and creamy texture. This is perhaps the simplest way to enjoy mackerel—simply marinated in ginger and lime and served with a bowl of crunchy cilantro slaw.

CHILE-LIME MACKEREL

2 to 3 fillets (300 g/10.6 oz) raw mackerel

1 tablespoon (6 g/0.2 oz) grated fresh ginger

1 small (5 g/0.2 oz) red chile pepper, finely chopped

1 clove garlic, minced

1 tablespoon (15 ml) fresh lime juice

2 tablespoons (30 ml) extra-virgin avocado oil

Salt and black pepper, to taste

CILANTRO SLAW

1 cup (70 g/2.5 oz) shredded green cabbage

1 cup (70 g/2.5 oz) shredded red cabbage

2 tablespoons (12 g/0.4 oz) chopped fresh cilantro or parsley

2 medium (30 g/1.1 oz) spring onions, chopped

2 tablespoons (30 ml) Blender Mayonnaise (page 199) or avocado oil mayonnaise

1 tablespoon (15 ml) extra-virgin olive oil

1 tablespoon (15 ml) fresh lime juice

Salt and black pepper, to taste

Optional: lime wedges and sliced fresh chiles, to serve

① To make the mackerel: Make 3 or 4 shallow diagonal slits in the skin of the mackerel fillets. In a small bowl, combine all of the remaining ingredients for the marinade. Place the mackerel fillets on a plate and drizzle over the marinade. Marinate in the fridge for 30 minutes or overnight.

② To make the slaw: Place the cabbage in a bowl and add the cilantro, spring onions, mayonnaise, olive oil, and lime juice. Mix to combine. Season with salt and pepper. Refrigerate while you cook the mackerel.

③ Preheat the oven to 320°F (160°C) fan assisted or 355°F (180°C) conventional. Place the mackerel fillets on a baking tray, skin-side up, lined with parchment paper. Transfer to the oven and bake for 15 to 20 minutes, turning the tray halfway, until cooked through. Remove from the oven and set aside.

④ Serve with the prepared slaw along with lime wedges and chiles, if using. Store in the fridge for up to 3 days.

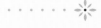 **FUN FACT**

Chiles contain capsaicin, the "spicy" molecule. By binding to the TRPV1 receptor, capsaicin can regulate your gut's nerve to help you poop if you're constipated.

NUTRITION FACTS PER SERVING:

Total carbs: 8.4 g	Fat: 54.2 g (of which saturated: 9.2 g)	SAT / MUFA / PUFA (%): 17, 61, 22
Fiber: 2.4 g	Calories: 636 kcal	Omega-6/3 ratio: 0.8 ☺
Net Carbs: 6 g	Macronutrient ratio: Calories from carbs (4%), protein (19%), fat (77%)	
Protein: 29.6 g		

DEVILED MACKEREL WITH FENNEL SLAW

Fans of paprika- and cayenne-tinged deviled eggs will fall in love with this summery dish. Mackerel gets doused in a spicy marinade and baked until tender, and then it's paired with a simple slaw of shaved fennel, sliced celery, and tons of fresh herbs. Skeptical about just how devilish this "deviled" mackerel really is? Check out the per-serving calorie content!

DEVILED MACKEREL

2 to 3 fillets (300 g/10.6 oz) raw mackerel

2 tablespoons (30 ml) extra-virgin avocado oil or ghee

1 teaspoon balsamic vinegar

1 teaspoon paprika

⅛ teaspoon cayenne pepper

Salt and black pepper, to taste

FENNEL SLAW

1 medium (200 g/7 oz) fennel bulb (fronds reserved for garnish)

1 medium (85 g/3 oz) celery stalk, sliced

½ small (30 g/1.1 oz) red onion, sliced

3 tablespoons (45 ml) extra-virgin olive oil

1 tablespoon (15 ml) fresh lemon juice

1 teaspoon fresh lemon zest

1 clove garlic, minced

2 tablespoons (8 g/0.4 oz) chopped fresh parsley, mint, and/or tarragon

Salt and black pepper, to taste

① To make the mackerel: Make 3 or 4 shallow diagonal slits in the skin of the mackerel fillets. In a small bowl, combine all of the remaining ingredients for the marinade. Place the mackerel fillets on a plate and drizzle over the marinade. Marinate in the fridge for 30 minutes or overnight.

② To make the slaw: Using a sharp knife or mandoline, thinly slice the fennel, or place it in a food processor and process using the slicing blade. Add to a bowl together with the remaining slaw ingredients and combine well.

③ Preheat the oven to 320°F (160°C) fan assisted or 355°F (180°C) conventional. Place the mackerel fillets, skin-side up, on a baking tray lined with parchment paper. Transfer to the oven and bake for 15 to 20 minutes, turning the tray halfway, until cooked through. Remove from the oven and set aside.

④ Serve with the prepared slaw. Store in the fridge for up to 3 days.

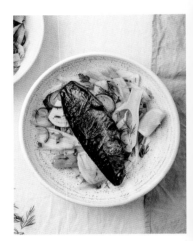

NUTRITION FACTS PER SERVING:

Total carbs: 12.4 g	Fat: 55.6 g (of which saturated: 9.4 g)	SAT / MUFA / PUFA (%): 17, 63, 20
Fiber: 4.8 g	Calories: 666 kcal	Omega-6/3 ratio: 1.0 ☺
Net Carbs: 7.6 g	Macronutrient ratio: Calories from carbs (5%), protein (18%), fat (77%)	
Protein: 30.1 g		

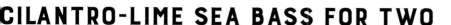

CILANTRO-LIME SEA BASS FOR TWO

This recipe tastes way more complicated than it actually is. Panfried seabass and crunchy steamed broccoli are easy to prepare; all that's left to do is to stir together the herbed dressing and spoon it over the finished meal. Consider making a double batch of the dressing; we're pretty sure you'll want to lavish it on just about anything! Be sure to finish your broccoli—numerous studies have shown that regularly consuming cruciferous vegetables, such as broccoli, is associated with reduced cancer risk.

SEA BASS & BROCCOLI

10.6 ounces (300 g) broccolini or small head broccoli, cut into florets

2 to 3 fillets (300 g/10.6 oz) sea bass

1 tablespoon (15 ml) extra-virgin avocado oil or ghee

Salt and black pepper, to taste

LIME-CORIANDER DRESSING

2 tablespoons (30 ml) fresh lime juice

6 tablespoons (90 ml) extra-virgin olive oil

1 tablespoon (8 g/0.3 oz) drained capers

1 clove garlic, crushed

1 teaspoon Dijon or yellow mustard

3 tablespoons (12 g/0.4 oz) chopped fresh cilantro

Salt and black pepper, to taste

1 tablespoon (15 ml) coconut aminos

Optional: chile flakes, to serve

① To make the sea bass & broccoli: Place the broccoli in a steamer filled with about 1½ cups (360 ml) of water, or place in a pot with a steamer colander on the bottom. Bring to a boil and cover with a lid. Cook over medium-high heat for 5 to 8 minutes, or until crisp-tender. Remove from the heat, remove the lid, and let the steam escape.

② Score the skin of the sea bass 3 times with a sharp knife to stop the skin from curling up while cooking. Grease a skillet with the avocado oil and add the sea bass, skin-side down. Cook for 3 to 4 minutes over medium heat until crisp and golden. Flip over and cook for 1 to 2 minutes, or until the flesh turns opaque. Season with salt and pepper.

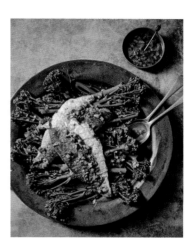

③ To make the dressing: Combine all the dressing ingredients in a small bowl. Serve the sea bass with the broccoli, and top with the dressing. Eat warm with a sprinkling of chile flakes or let cool and refrigerate for up to 3 days.

NUTRITION FACTS PER SERVING:

Total carbs: 12.7 g	Fat: 53.8 g (of which saturated: 7.7 g)	SAT / MUFA / PUFA (%): 14, 73, 13
Fiber: 4.4 g	Calories: 652 kcal	Omega-6/3 ratio: 2.9
Net Carbs: 8.3 g	Macronutrient ratio: Calories from carbs (6%), protein (13%), fat (81%)	
Protein: 33 g		

BACON-WRAPPED SCALLOPS WITH AVO-AIOLI DIP

This is the easiest-ever dish to prepare, and all it takes is a handful of high-quality ingredients. Just wrap juicy scallops in crispy bacon slices, pop them in the oven until the bacon is crisp and the scallops are cooked through, and serve with a MUFA-packed avocado aioli for dipping. A simple bowl of dressed greens rounds out this light, romantic meal beautifully.

SCALLOPS

1.3 pounds (600 g) scallops
(12 to 16 depending on size)

6.4 ounces (180 g) bacon
or pancetta

1 tablespoon (15 ml) extra-virgin
avocado oil or ghee

Salt and black pepper, to taste

1 tablespoon (4 g/0.2 oz)
chopped fresh herbs, such as
parsley or chives

AVO-AIOLI DIP

½ cup (120 ml) Blender Mayonnaise
(page 199) or avocado oil
mayonnaise

1 clove garlic, minced

1 tablespoon (15 ml) fresh
lemon juice

½ medium (75 g/2.7 oz) avocado

Optional: side salad of your choice,
to serve

① Preheat the oven to 400°F (200°C) fan assisted or 425°F (220°C) conventional. Line a baking dish with parchment paper.

② To make the scallops: Using a paper kitchen towel, pat dry the scallops to remove excess moisture. Wrap a slice of bacon around each scallop and secure with a toothpick. Arrange the scallops in a single layer on the baking tray. Brush with the avocado oil and season to taste with salt and pepper. Place in the oven and bake for 10 to 15 minutes, until the bacon is crisped up and the scallops are cooked through (extra-large and jumbo scallops will take longer to cook). Remove from the oven and let rest for 5 minutes. (Alternatively, you could cook the seasoned, bacon-wrapped scallops in a hot nonstick pan for about 2 to 3 minutes per side.)

③ To make the dip: Place all of the avo-aioli ingredients in a blender and process until smooth. Serve the scallops with the dip and, optionally, any side salad of your choice.

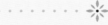 **FUN FACT**

Scallops are among the world's richest sources of taurine, which can reduce blood pressure, while pork and avocado oil are rich in MUFA. Garlic is also widely reported to have cardioprotective properties. This means that this "indulgent" treat is a treat for your ticker, too.

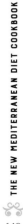

NUTRITION FACTS PER SERVING (3 TO 4 SCALLOPS + ¼ CUP [60 ML] AVO-AIOLI DIP):

Total carbs: 7.2 g	Fat: 34.3 g (of which saturated: 8.7 g)	SAT / MUFA / PUFA (%): 25, 58, 17
Fiber: 1.4 g	Calories: 465 kcal	Omega-6: 4.7 g
Net Carbs: 5.8 g	Macronutrient ratio: Calories from carbs (5%), protein (28%), fat (67%)	
Protein: 32.4 g		

RAISED OCTOPUS WITH WHITE WINE & FENNEL

Octopus is a seafood staple in Greek cuisine: in fact, this recipe is based on a traditional Greek preparation. No need for complicated ingredients here: just a few herbs and spices, and a little vinegar and white wine, are enough to produce juicy, tender flesh. Serve this tapas-style at a late summer dinner al fresco surrounded by salads of fresh low-carb veggies.

medium (2 pounds/900 g) raw octopus

tablespoons (45 ml) white wine vinegar

cup (120 ml) dry white wine

½ teaspoons fennel seeds

bay leaves

RESSING

cup (180 ml) extra-virgin olive oil

cup (60 ml) fresh lemon juice

tablespoons (8 g/0.3 oz) chopped fresh parsley

teaspoon chile flakes or teaspoon ground black pepper

① Rub the octopus with salt and wash under cold running water to get rid of slime and other impurities. Remove the beak.

② Place the octopus in a large saucepan, along with the white wine vinegar, white wine, fennel seeds, and bay leaves. Bring to a boil, then lower the heat to a very low simmer, cover tightly with a lid, and cook over low heat for 50 to 55 minutes. There is no need to add water, as the octopus will release juices as it cooks, but be sure the lid is on tightly to prevent the moisture from evaporating. Do not add any salt: it is already salty from sea water. The octopus is done when a knife inserted into the thickest part yields easily. Transfer to a chopping board and let cool slightly before slicing.

③ Meanwhile, keep cooking the stock until reduced by half. Remove from the heat and let cool completely. When cool, strain through a sieve and discard the spices.

④ To make the dressing: Whisk the stock with the olive oil, lemon juice, parsley, and chile flakes.

⑤ Cut the tentacles off, slice the head into thick pieces, and slice the tentacles. Toss it with the prepared dressing. Serve with any side salad. To store, refrigerate for up to 3 days.

NUTRITION FACTS PER SERVING:

otal carbs: 7.3 g	Fat: 43 g (of which saturated: 6.1 g)	SAT / MUFA / PUFA (%): 14, 76, 10
iber: 0.4 g	Calories: 576 kcal	Omega-6: 4.2 g
et Carbs: 6.9 g	Macronutrient ratio: Calories from carbs	
rotein: 33.8 g	(5%), protein (25%), fat (70%)	

SEAFOOD CAULI-PAELLA

Inspired by traditional Spanish paella, a one-pot smorgasbord of rice, seafood, sausage, and vegetables, this low-carb skillet meal is made with three types of seafood plus a saffron- and herb-infused cauli-rice. It's actually much easier to make than the original version, but it's just as satisfying—and way healthier. All that seafood promotes healthy brain function: in fact, studies now show that omega-3s can even protect against sleep deprivation–induced memory impairments.

Pinch of saffron

¼ cup (60 ml) water

FISH & SEAFOOD

2 fillets (300 g/10.6 oz) wild salmon

5.3 ounces (150 g) raw prawns

5.3 ounces (150 g) squid rings

1 tablespoon (15 ml) fresh lemon juice

Pinch of salt and black pepper

2 tablespoons (30 ml) extra-virgin avocado oil or ghee, divided

PAELLA

1 medium (680 g/1.5 lb) cauliflower

3 tablespoons (45 ml) extra-virgin avocado oil or ghee

½ small (30 g/1.1 oz) red onion

4 cloves garlic, minced

¼ cup (60 ml) chicken stock

2 tablespoons (30 g/1.1 oz) tomato paste

1 teaspoon paprika

¼ to ½ teaspoon cayenne pepper

¼ cup (15 g/0.5 oz) chopped fresh parsley

6 tablespoons (90 ml) extra-virgin olive oil

Chile pepper flakes, to taste

① First, soak the saffron in ¼ cup (60 ml) of water.

② To make the fish & seafood: Drizzle the salmon, prawns, and squid rings with the lemon juice, then season with salt and pepper. Heat a skillet with 1 tablespoon (15 ml) of the avocado oil and add the salmon, skin-side down. Cook over medium heat for 3 to 4 minutes per side, until browned and cooked through. Remove from the pan and set aside.

③ Grease the same pan in which you cooked the salmon with the remaining 1 tablespoon (15 ml) avocado oil and add the prawns and squid rings. Cook for 2 to 3 minutes, until opaque, and then transfer to a bowl and keep warm.

④ To make the paella: Run the cauliflower florets through a hand grater or food processor with the S or the grating blade. Process until the florets resemble grains of rice. Grease a large skillet with the avocado oil. Add the onion and cook over medium-high heat for about 5 minutes. Add garlic and cook for 1 minute. Add the cauliflower rice, stock, soaked saffron with its liquid, tomato paste, paprika, and cayenne pepper. Cook until the cauliflower is crisp-tender, about 5 to 7 minutes.

⑤ Return the cooked shrimp, squid, and flaked salmon to the skillet and cook to heat through for a minute or two. Remove from the heat and add most of the parsley. Drizzle with the olive oil and garnish with more parsley and chile flakes. Eat warm or store in the fridge for up to 4 days.

NUTRITION FACTS PER SERVING:

Total carbs: 13 g	Fat: 44 g (of which saturated: 6.4 g)	SAT / MUFA / PUFA (%): 14, 72, 14
Fiber: 4.1 g	Calories: 564 kcal	Omega-6/3 ratio: 1.8 ☺
Net Carbs: 8.9 g	Macronutrient ratio: Calories from carbs (6%), protein (23%), fat (71%)	
Protein: 31.7 g		

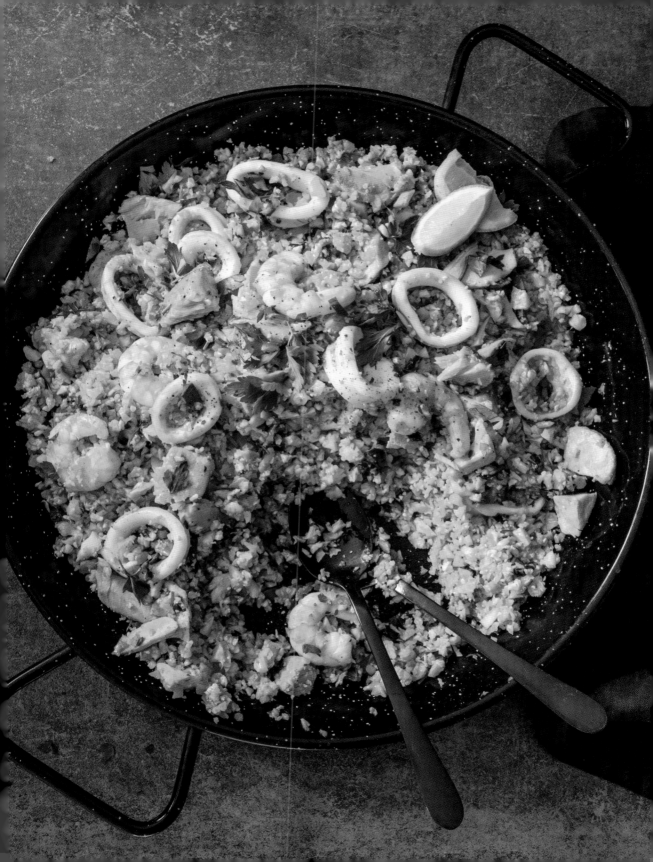

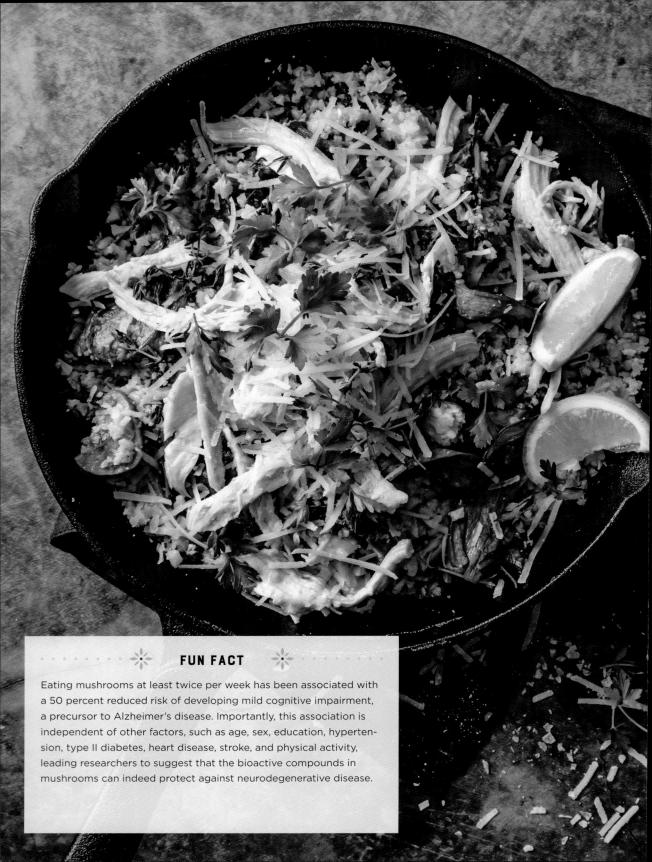

FUN FACT

Eating mushrooms at least twice per week has been associated with a 50 percent reduced risk of developing mild cognitive impairment, a precursor to Alzheimer's disease. Importantly, this association is independent of other factors, such as age, sex, education, hypertension, type II diabetes, heart disease, stroke, and physical activity, leading researchers to suggest that the bioactive compounds in mushrooms can indeed protect against neurodegenerative disease.

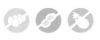

WILD MUSHROOM CHICKEN RISOTTO

"Regular" risotto is made with starchy Arborio rice, so it's off-limits if you're following a keto diet. But this keto-friendly adaptation is every bit as satisfying. Our creamy mushroom risotto is made with earthy porcini mushrooms, tender chicken, plenty of shaved Pecorino Romano, and extra-virgin olive oil to add lots of nutritious fats. Make it for your next date night: it simply can't fail to impress.

1 cup (30 g/1.1 oz) wild dried porcini mushrooms, or 2 cups (100 g/3.5 oz) fresh wild mushrooms

1 cup (240 ml) hot water

½ medium (360 g/12.7 oz) cauliflower

1 medium (200 g/7 oz) chicken breast, skinless and boneless

Salt and black pepper, to taste

3 tablespoons (45 ml) extra-virgin avocado oil or ghee, divided

½ small (30 g/1.1 oz) red onion

1 clove garlic, minced

1 cup (30 g/1.1 oz) fresh spinach, chopped

½ cup plus 2 tablespoons (57 g/ 2 oz) grated or flaked Pecorino Romano, divided

2 tablespoons (8 g/0.3 oz) chopped fresh herbs, such as parsley, basil, chives, and/or thyme

1½ teaspoons fresh lemon juice

2 tablespoons (30 ml) extra-virgin olive oil

① Place the dried mushrooms in a bowl and add the hot water. Soak for at least 30 minutes to soften, and then drain.

② Run the cauliflower through a hand grater or food processor with the S or the grating blade. Process until the florets resemble grains of rice. Set aside.

③ Tenderize the chicken breast with a rolling pin or a meat tenderizer to achieve an even thickness. Season with a pinch of salt and pepper.

④ Heat a large skillet with 1 tablespoon (15 ml) of the avocado oil over medium-high heat and add the chicken. Depending on the thickness, cook for 4 to 6 minutes per side. Transfer to a chopping board and let cool before slicing.

⑤ Grease the same skillet in which you cooked the chicken with the remaining 2 tablespoons (30 ml) avocado oil. Add the onion and cook for 3 to 5 minutes. Add the garlic and cook for 1 minute. Add the cauli-rice and cook for 5 to 7 minutes or until crisp-tender. Add the soaked mushrooms, spinach, cheese (reserve some for topping), herbs, and lemon juice. Add back the chicken, cook to heat through, and season with salt and pepper.

⑥ Remove from the heat and drizzle with the olive oil. Sprinkle with more herbs and add the remaining cheese. Serve warm, or let it cool down and refrigerate for up to 4 days.

NUTRITION FACTS PER SERVING:

Total carbs: 13.9 g	Fat: 45.4 g (of which saturated: 9.7 g)	SAT / MUFA / PUFA (%): 21, 67, 12
Fiber: 4.8 g	Calories: 604 kcal	Omega-6: 4.6 g
Net Carbs: 9.1 g	Macronutrient ratio: Calories from carbs (6%), protein (25%), fat (69%)	
Protein: 37.9 g		

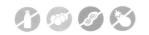

SERVINGS:	HANDS-ON TIME:	OVERALL TIME:
4 (8 skewers)	20 minutes	20 minutes + marinating

KARL'S CHICKEN SOUVLAKI

(CONTRIBUTOR: CHRIS ROMANKO)

Souvlaki has been one of the most popular street foods in Greece for centuries, making these chicken skewers, contributed by Chris Romanko, timeless. One night, Chris's two-year-old infant son, Karl, had a seizure. Soon, Karl was having eighty seizures a day. Chris recalls, "He was hospitalized a number of times and treated with different medications, but nothing helped." Then Karl began a ketogenic diet. Keto saved Karl, and Chris and her partner "are overjoyed to have our son back."

MARINATED CHICKEN

1.5 pounds (680 g) raw chicken breasts, skinless and boneless, cut into 2-inch (5 cm) chunks

½ cup (120 ml) extra-virgin avocado oil, divided

¼ cup (60 ml) fresh lemon juice

½ teaspoon salt

½ teaspoon black pepper

1 small (60 g/2.1 oz) red onion, roughly chopped

¼ cup (16 g) chopped fresh herbs, such as oregano, mint, thyme, parsley, tarragon, and/or rosemary

LEMON DRESSING

¼ cup (60 ml) extra-virgin olive oil

1 tablespoon (15 ml) fresh lemon juice

1 tablespoon (4 g/0.2 oz) chopped fresh herbs of your choice, as above

① To make the chicken: Place the chicken chunks in a bowl. Add all the remaining ingredients except for 2 tablespoons (30 ml) of avocado oil. Stir to coat the meat in the marinade. Cover with aluminum foil and refrigerate for at least 2 hours, or for up to 24 hours.

② When you're ready to cook, thread the chicken chunks onto skewers, 4 per skewer. You can reuse the marinade for another batch. Store it in the fridge for up to 1 day. Heat a large griddle pan (or regular pan greased with the remaining avocado oil) over medium-high heat. Once hot, add the skewers in a single layer and cook for 8 to 10 minutes, turning with a fork (or your fingers, if using wooden skewers), until cooked through and browned on all sides.

③ To make the dressing: Whisk the olive oil and lemon juice in a small bowl until emulsified.

④ Drizzle the dressing over the skewers and sprinkle with the fresh herbs. Serve with a bowl of Taverna-Style Greek Salad (page 82), Fennel Tzatziki (page 72), or Upgraded Baba Ghanoush (page 78).

THE NEW MEDITERRANEAN DIET COOKBOOK

NUTRITION FACTS PER SERVING (2 SKEWERS):

Total carbs: 1.3 g	Fat: 28.5 g (of which saturated: 4 g)	SAT / MUFA / PUFA (%): 14, 71, 15
Fiber: 0.3 g	Calories: 421 kcal	Omega-6: 3.2 g
Net Carbs: 1 g	Macronutrient ratio: Calories from carbs (1%), protein (37%), fat (62%)	
Protein: 38.4 g		

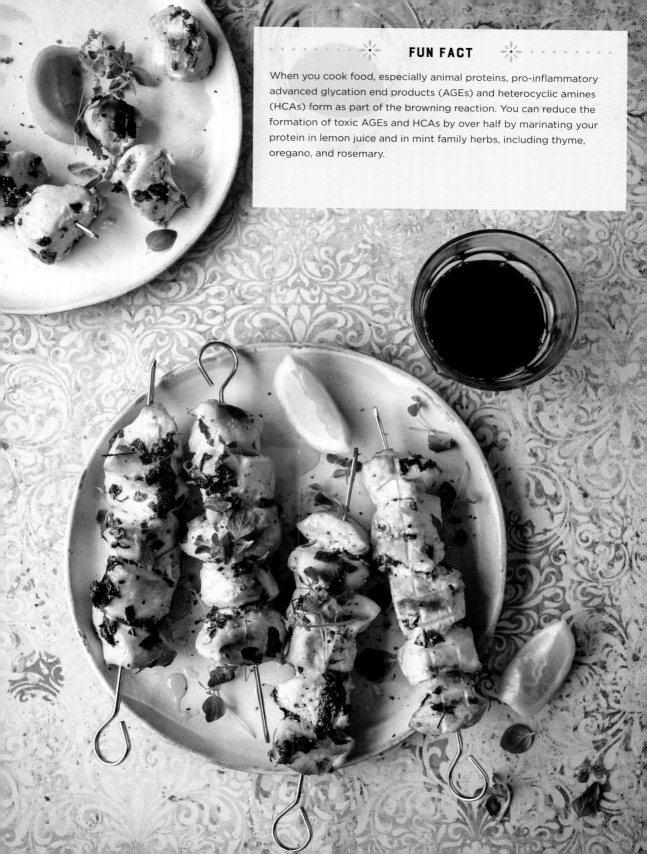

FUN FACT

When you cook food, especially animal proteins, pro-inflammatory advanced glycation end products (AGEs) and heterocyclic amines (HCAs) form as part of the browning reaction. You can reduce the formation of toxic AGEs and HCAs by over half by marinating your protein in lemon juice and in mint family herbs, including thyme, oregano, and rosemary.

SCIENCY LIVER SAUTÉ SKILLET

(CONTRIBUTOR: DR. ELENA GROSS)

This recipe was contributed by Dr. Elena Gross, one of the world's leading experts on migraines. According to Dr. Gross, ketogenic diets plus particular micronutrients such as riboflavin, coenzyme Q_{10}, and magnesium can help prevent migraines. If you suffer from migraines, this one-skillet dish could help: Liver is the world's best source of riboflavin and is also an amazing source of coenzyme Q_{10}, while spinach is among the richest vegetable sources of both coenzyme Q_{10} and magnesium.

CHICKEN LIVERS

1.3 pounds (600 g) raw chicken livers, cleaned

1 tablespoon (15 ml) red wine vinegar or apple cider vinegar

3 tablespoons (45 ml) extra-virgin avocado oil or ghee, divided

Salt and black pepper, to taste

2 cloves garlic, minced

2 tablespoons (6 g/0.2 oz) chopped fresh sage

1 cup (70 g/2.5 oz) chopped white mushrooms

5 ounces (142 g) fresh spinach or equivalent amount of frozen, thawed, and drained spinach

¼ cup (60 ml) extra-virgin olive oil, to drizzle

GRAVY

¾ cup (180 ml) chicken stock

4 egg yolks

Salt and black pepper, to taste

1 tablespoon (3 g/0.1 oz) chopped fresh chives

Optional: ¼ teaspoon smoked paprika

TO SERVE

Green Cauli-Mash (page 157) or Cauli-Rice (page 166)

① To make the chicken livers: Cut the livers into chunks and cut out any tough parts. Place in a bowl filled with filtered water and the vinegar. Refrigerate for at least 6 hours or overnight. This will remove the strong scent and will help achieve a smooth taste. When ready to cook, drain the livers and pat dry with a paper towel.

② Heat a large skillet greased with 1 tablespoon (15 ml) of the avocado oil over medium-high heat. Add the chicken livers, preferably in batches, and cook for 4 to 6 minutes. Season with salt and pepper and use a slotted spoon to transfer to a plate when done. Clean the pan with a paper towel and then grease with the remaining 2 tablespoons (30 ml) avocado oil. Add the garlic and sage and cook over medium heat for 1 to 2 minutes, until fragrant. Add the mushrooms and cook for 5 to 7 minutes, until tender. Finally, add the spinach in two batches and cook until wilted, about 1 minute. Return the livers to the skillet and heat through for just a minute. Remove from the heat and drizzle with the olive oil.

③ To make the gravy: In a small saucepan, bring the chicken stock to a boil. In a mixing bowl, whisk the egg yolks with a pinch of salt and pepper. To temper the egg yolks, add the hot stock, 1 tablespoon (15 ml) at a time, while whisking. When all of the stock has been used, pour the egg-stock mixture back into the skillet. Gently heat for 1 to 2 minutes, whisking constantly, until it thickens slightly. Pour it into the skillet over the livers.

④ Garnish with the chives and, optionally, smoked paprika. Serve with cauli-mash or cauli-rice.

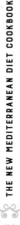
THE NEW MEDITERRANEAN DIET COOKBOOK

NUTRITION FACTS PER SERVING:

Total carbs: 4.3 g	Fat: 36.9 g (of which saturated: 7.5 g)	SAT / MUFA / PUFA (%): 20, 67, 13
Fiber: 1.1 g	Calories: 473 kcal	Omega-6: 3.9 g
Net Carbs: 3.2 g	Macronutrient ratio: Calories from carbs (3%), protein (26%), fat (71%)	
Protein: 30.7 g		

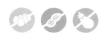

CREAMY TARRAGON CHICKEN WITH CABBAGE & CRISPY BACON

Here, tender chicken is cooked in a creamy lemon-tarragon sauce and served with crunchy cabbage noodles and crispy bacon. It's a real crowd-pleaser that you can have on the table in under 30 minutes.

MARINADE & CHICKEN

2 tablespoons (30 ml) extra-virgin avocado oil

Zest from ½ lemon

Salt and black pepper, to taste

2 large (500 g/1.1 pounds) chicken or turkey thighs, cut into chunks

SAUCE

2 tablespoons (30 ml) extra-virgin avocado oil

½ small (30 g/1.1 oz) red onion, diced

1 cup (70 g/2.5 oz) sliced white or brown mushrooms

1 cup (240 ml) chicken stock

½ cup (120 ml) goat's cream or heavy whipping cream

1 tablespoon (30 ml) fresh lemon juice

2 tablespoons (6 g/0.2 oz) chopped fresh tarragon

Salt and black pepper, to taste

CABBAGE

3 ounces (85 g) bacon slices, cut into thin strips

¾ to 1 cup (180 to 240 ml) water, divided

2 tablespoons (30 ml) extra-virgin avocado oil

1 small head (600 g/1.3 lb) savoy cabbage, core removed, sliced into noodles

Pinch of salt and black pepper

① To make the marinade & chicken: Combine the avocado oil, lemon zest, salt, and pepper in a small bowl. Add the chicken to a separate bowl. Pour over the marinade and refrigerate for 2 hours or overnight.

② To make the sauce: Heat a skillet greased with the avocado oil over medium heat. Add the onion and cook for 3 to 5 minutes. Add the chicken thighs with the marinade and cook for about 8 minutes, stirring occasionally. Add the mushrooms and cook for 3 to 5 minutes. Pour in the chicken stock, bring to a boil, and simmer for 5 minutes. Add the cream, reduce the heat, and cook for 5 minutes. Finally, add the lemon juice and tarragon, stir to combine, and season with salt and pepper to taste. Remove from the heat and cover with a lid to keep warm.

③ To make the cabbage: Place the bacon pieces in a hot pan with about ½ cup (120 ml) of the water. Cook over medium-high heat for 5 to 8 minutes until the fat is rendered and the bacon is lightly crisped up. Remove from the heat and use a slotted spoon to transfer to a plate. Grease the same pan in which you cooked the bacon with the avocado oil and add the sliced cabbage. Add the remaining ¼ to ½ cup (60 to 120 ml) water and season with a pinch of salt and pepper. Cover with a lid and cook over medium-low heat for 8 to 12 minutes, or until the cabbage is crisp-tender. Remove from the heat and stir in the bacon. Serve with the creamy tarragon chicken. To store, let cool and refrigerate for up to 4 days.

NUTRITION FACTS PER SERVING:

Total carbs: 11.8 g	Fat: 44.3 g (of which saturated: 13.5 g)	SAT / MUFA / PUFA (%): 30, 55, 15
Fiber: 5.1 g	Calories: 572 kcal	Omega-6: 4.6 g
Net Carbs: 6.7 g	Macronutrient ratio: Calories from carbs	
Protein: 33 g	(5%), protein (24%), fat (71%)	

FIERCE MEATBALL ZOODLE BOLOGNESE

(CONTRIBUTOR: SUPERMAX!)

Juicy, kid-friendly meatballs in an herby tomato sauce are served on a bed of twirly zucchini noodles and topped with Pecorino Romano shavings. This recipe is courtesy of a very special contributor: In 2011, when he was just four years old, Max Wilford was diagnosed with a serious type of brain tumor. But Max has thrived on a therapeutic ketogenic diet. His story inspired the MaxLove Project, a nonprofit with a mission to increase quality of life for children surviving cancer, which includes a ketogenic diet as a facet of their *Fierce Foods* nutrition program. Max says, "I don't eat spaghetti, but I *love* zoodles. With meatballs and tons of cheese too, *Fierce* Meatball Zoodle Bolognese is awesome sauce!"

MEATBALLS

1.1 pounds (500 g) grass-fed ground beef (15% fat)

½ teaspoon salt

¼ teaspoon black pepper

2 large egg yolks

3 tablespoons (21 g/0.8 oz) flax meal

1 teaspoon dried Italian herbs or 1 tablespoon (4 g/0.2 oz) chopped fresh herbs, such as thyme, oregano, and basil

2 tablespoons (30 ml) extra-virgin avocado oil

BOLOGNESE SAUCE

1 small (60 g/2.1 oz) red onion

1 teaspoon (2 g) chopped fresh rosemary

2 cloves garlic, minced

1 medium (60 g/2.1 oz) celery stalk, sliced

1 cup (240 ml) canned peeled tomatoes

1 tablespoon (15 ml) unsweetened tomato purée

1 cup (240 ml) chicken stock or bone broth

1 teaspoon dried oregano

2 bay leaves

TO SERVE

2 tablespoons (30 ml) extra-virgin olive oil

3 medium (600 g/1.3 lb) zucchini, spiralized and core chopped

½ cup (57 g/2 oz) flaked Pecorino Romano

Pinch of salt and black pepper, to taste

Fresh basil leaves, to taste

① To make the meatballs: Combine all the ingredients except the avocado oil in a bowl. Using your hands, form the mixture into 20 meatballs (about 28 g/1 oz each). Grease a large skillet with the oil. Once hot, add the meatballs in a single layer. Cook for 2 minutes per side, turning with a fork until browned on all sides and cooked through. Remove from the heat.

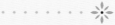 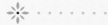

FUN FACT

Max loves *Star Wars,* history, his puppy, Zeus, and cooking. He's a whiz at "ketofying" Italian, Indian, and Japanese foods, and his favorite bread is Martina's focaccia (page 179), which he makes into grilled cheese sandwiches soaked with grass-fed goat's butter.

NUTRITION FACTS PER SERVING (5 MEATBALLS • SAUCE AND ZOODLES):

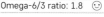

Total carbs: 12.3 g	Fat: 48.9 g (of which saturated: 15.3 g)	SAT / MUFA / PUFA (%): 31, 57, 12
Fiber: 5.1 g	Calories: 616 kcal	Omega-6/3 ratio: 1.8 ☺
Net Carbs: 7.2 g	Macronutrient ratio: Calories from carbs (5%), protein (22%), fat (73%)	
Protein: 32.9 g		

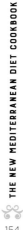

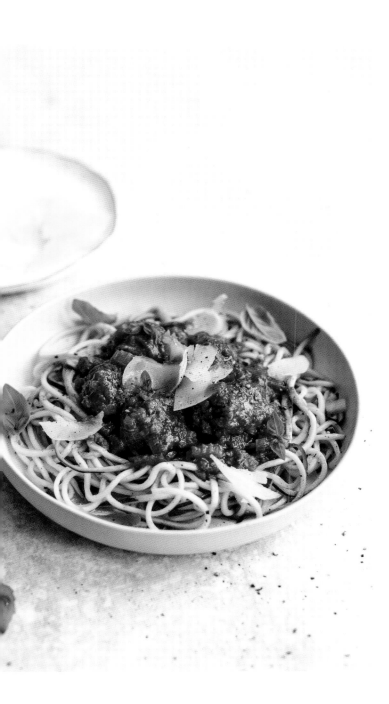

② To make the sauce: To the skillet where you cooked the meatballs, add the onion and cook for about 3 to 5 minutes. Add the rosemary and garlic and cook for 1 minute. Add the remaining ingredients for the sauce and bring to a boil. Simmer over medium-low heat for about 10 minutes or until the sauce is reduced by half. Add back the meatballs and heat through. Take off the heat and set aside.

③ To serve: Grease a large pan with the olive oil and add the zucchini. Cook over medium-high heat for 2 to 3 minutes, then remove from the heat and set aside. You can also serve the "zoodles" raw and simply drizzle some olive oil over them.

④ Place the "zoodles" into serving bowls and top with the sauce and meatballs. Garnish with the Pecorino Romano, salt, pepper, and basil. The meatballs can be stored in the fridge for up to 4 days or frozen for up to 3 months. The zucchini noodles are best prepared fresh, but you can store them in the fridge for up to 1 day.

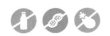
RUMINATION-FREE STEAK WITH CREAMY BÉARNAISE SAUCE

(CONTRIBUTOR: GUY WINCH)

This juicy pan-seared steak served with steamed broccoli and a generous dollop of creamy, dairy-free béarnaise sauce was contributed by Guy Winch, a psychologist and leading voice in the science of emotional health. His TED Talks have received more than 20 million views: one of our favorites is called "How to turn off work thoughts in your free time." After you enjoy this beefy, vitamin B_{12}– and zinc-packed meal, we recommend taking a few minutes out to watch Guy's brilliant talk on how to avoid "ruminating," so you don't end up turning into a "thought cow."

STEAK & VEG

2 lean beef steaks (300 g/10.6 oz) such as fillet, rump, sirloin, flank, or skirt

1 tablespoon (15 ml) extra-virgin avocado oil or ghee

Pinch of salt and black pepper

10.6 ounces (300 g) broccolini or 1 small broccoli, cut into florets

1 cup (240 ml) water

BÉARNAISE SAUCE

½ small (30 g/1.1 oz) onion, roughly chopped

2 tablespoons (6 g/0.2 oz) chopped fresh tarragon or other herbs of your choice, divided

2 tablespoons (30 ml) apple cider vinegar

1 tablespoon (15 ml) water

2 egg yolks

1 tablespoon (15 ml) fresh lemon juice

¼ teaspoon Dijon or yellow mustard

¼ cup (60 ml) extra-virgin olive oil or ghee

Salt and black pepper, to taste

① To make the steaks: Grease both sides of the steaks with the avocado oil and season with salt and pepper. Fry in a hot dry pan over high heat for 2 to 4 minutes on each side to seal in the juices. When you see the edges start to brown, it's time to flip the steaks over. Reduce the heat to medium. Continue to cook for 4 minutes (rare), 7 minutes (medium), or 11 minutes (well done). Remove the steaks from the pan and allow them to rest in a warm place for a few minutes.

② While the steak is resting, place the broccoli in a steamer (or a saucepan with a steamer colander inside) and fill with about 1 cup (240 ml) of water. Bring to a boil, cover with a lid, and steam for about 5 minutes, or until crisp-tender. Remove the lid and let the steam escape.

③ To make the béarnaise sauce: Place the onion, half of the tarragon, vinegar, and water in a medium saucepan. Cook over medium heat for 3 minutes, or until the liquid is reduced to just 2 tablespoons (30 ml). Strain, discard the solids, and set aside until cool.

④ Fill a medium saucepan with 1 cup (240 ml) of water and bring to a boil. Mix the egg yolks with the lemon juice and mustard in a heatproof bowl. Add the cooled vinegar mixture; place the bowl over the saucepan filled with water. The water should not touch the bottom of the bowl. Mix continuously until the sauce starts to thicken. Slowly pour the olive oil into the mixture until thick and creamy, stirring constantly.

⑤ Remove from the heat, add the remaining tarragon, and season with salt and pepper. Serve warm with the steak and steamed broccoli.

NUTRITION FACTS PER SERVING:

Total carbs: 12 g	Fat: 46.2 g (of which saturated: 8.8 g)	SAT / MUFA / PUFA (%): 19, 70, 11
Fiber: 4.1 g	Calories: 616 kcal	Omega-6: 4.2 g
Net Carbs: 7.9 g	Macronutrient ratio: Calories from carbs	
Protein: 41.2 g	(5%), protein (27%), fat (68%)	

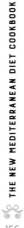

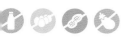

PORK MEDALLIONS WITH GREEN CAULI-MASH AND GRAVY

These pan-roasted medallions are served with a spinach-spiked cauli-mash instead of potatoes and a mushroom gravy. Among non-fish animal proteins, pork has the most Mediterranean fat profile. There are 25 percent more monounsaturated than saturated fats in pork.

GREEN CAULI-MASH

1 medium head (600 g/1.3 lb) cauliflower, cut into florets

⅓ cup (80 ml) extra-virgin olive oil or ghee

Salt and black pepper, to taste

4 cups (120 g/4.2 oz) fresh spinach or equivalent amount of frozen, thawed, and drained spinach, chopped

PORK & GRAVY

1.3 pounds (600 g) pork tenderloin, cut into 1-inch (2.5 cm) medallions

Salt and black pepper, to taste

2 tablespoons (30 ml) extra-virgin avocado oil or ghee, divided

½ medium (50 g/1.8 oz) red onion, sliced

2 cloves garlic, minced

2 tablespoons (6 g/0.2 oz) chopped fresh sage or rosemary

4 brown mushrooms (45 g/1.6 oz), sliced

2 tablespoons (30 ml) fresh lemon juice

½ cup (120 ml) chicken stock or bone broth

2 tablespoons (30 ml) extra-virgin olive oil

Optional: chopped fresh herbs, for garnish

① To make the mash: Place the cauliflower florets in a steamer filled with 1 cup (240 ml) water. Cook for about 10 minutes, until tender. Remove from the heat and place in a blender with the olive oil and salt and pepper to taste. Process until smooth, then stir in the spinach while still hot. The heat from the mash will soften the spinach.

② To make the pork: Season the sliced pork medallions with salt and pepper. Heat a large pan greased with 1 tablespoon (15 ml) of the avocado oil over medium-high heat. Add the medallions and cook for 3 to 4 minutes per side. Transfer to a plate and keep warm.

③ To make the gravy: Grease the same pan with the remaining 1 tablespoon (15 ml) avocado oil. Add the onion and cook for about 5 minutes. Add the garlic and herbs and cook for 1 minute. Add the mushrooms and cook for 5 minutes, until tender. Add the lemon juice and chicken stock and bring

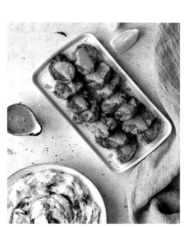

to a boil. Cook for 1 to 2 minutes, then remove from the heat. Pour the mixture into a tall, narrow plastic beaker or blender cup, add the olive oil, and use an immersion blender to process until creamy. Season to taste.

④ Serve the medallions with the cauli-mash and the gravy. Garnish with fresh herbs, if using. To store, refrigerate for up to 4 days.

NUTRITION FACTS PER SERVING (PORK + ABOUT 1 CUP [200 G/7 OZ] CAULI-MASH AND ¼ CUP [60 ML] GRAVY):

Total carbs: 11.2 g
Fiber: 4.1 g
Net Carbs: 7.1 g
Protein: 36.4 g

Fat: 36.2 g (of which saturated: 5.8 g)
Calories: 509 kcal
Macronutrient ratio: Calories from carbs (6%), protein (29%), fat (65%)

SAT / MUFA / PUFA (%): 16, 72, 12
Omega-6: 3.5 g

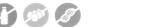

MOROCCAN LAMB TAGINE

Banish cold-weather blues with this Middle Eastern–style casserole: It combines melt-in-your-mouth lamb with warming Moroccan spices, eggplant and cauliflower (they're flavor sponges!), olives, and fresh herbs. Lamb is the richest source of conjugated linoleic acid, a healthy fat that is associated with lowered risks of heart disease, cancer, type II diabetes, and obesity.

¼ cup (60 ml) extra-virgin avocado oil or ghee

1 small (60 g/2.1 oz) red onion, chopped

¼ cup (15 g/0.5 oz) chopped fresh parsley or cilantro, stalks and leaves separated

2 cloves garlic, minced

1.1 pounds (500 g) stewing lamb, such as leg or shoulder, cut into 2-inch (5 cm) chunks

Salt and black pepper, to taste

¼ teaspoon cinnamon

1 teaspoon ground turmeric

4 teaspoons (10 g/0.4 oz) Harissa Spice Mix (page 198)

2 tablespoons (30 ml) unsweetened tomato paste

2 cups (480 ml) bone broth or chicken stock

1 small (250 g/8.8 oz) eggplant, cut into cubes

½ medium head (350 g/12.4 oz) cauliflower, cut into small florets

5 tablespoons (80 g/2.8 oz) coconut butter

½ cup (50 g/1.8 oz) pitted Kalamata olives

① Heat a large pot greased with the avocado oil over medium-high heat. Add the onion and cook for about 5 minutes. Chop the parsley stalks and add to the pot together with the minced garlic. Cook for 1 minute and add the lamb. Season with salt and pepper and cook until browned on all sides. Add the spices, tomato paste, and bone broth. Bring to a boil, cover with a lid, and reduce the heat to medium-low. Cook until the lamb is tender, about 1 hour 30 minutes. After about 1 hour and 10 minutes of cooking, add the eggplant and cauliflower. Stir to combine and cover with a lid.

② When the lamb and vegetables are tender, stir in the coconut butter and cook for 1 minute. Remove from the heat and stir in the olives and parsley leaves. Season to taste. To store, refrigerate for up to 4 days or freeze for up to 3 months.

 FUN FACT

Some studies have shown that daily intake of 3.2 grams or more of conjugated linoleic acid (CLA), a fatty acid found in grass-fed beef and lamb, reduces body fat in overweight people.

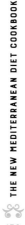
NUTRITION FACTS PER SERVING:

Total carbs: 16.9 g	Fat: 49.1 g (of which saturated: 21.8 g)	SAT / MUFA / PUFA (%): 44, 49, 7
Fiber: 8.1 g	Calories: 614 kcal	Omega-6: 2.4 g
Net Carbs: 8.8 g	Macronutrient ratio: Calories from carbs (6%), protein (20%), fat (74%)	
Protein: 29.3 g		

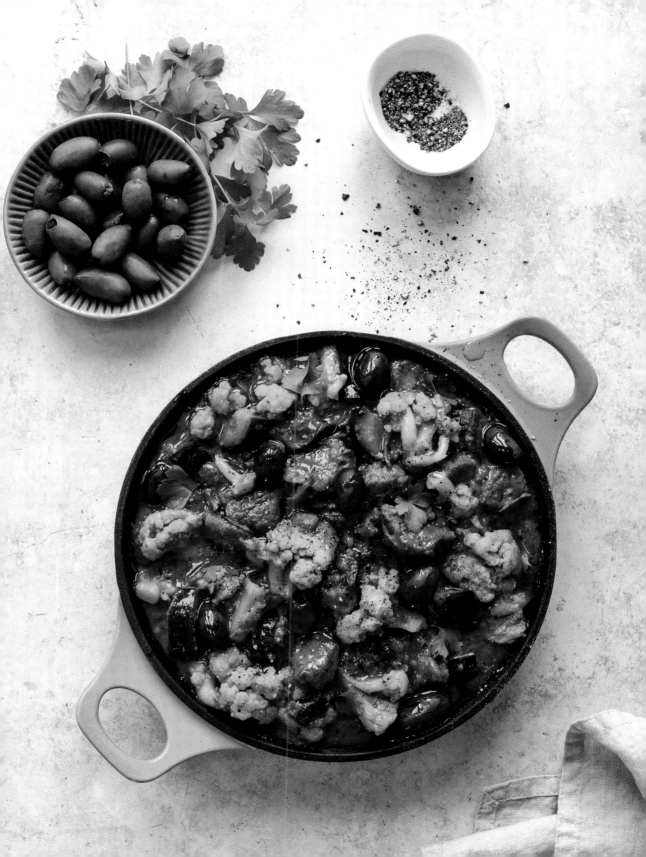

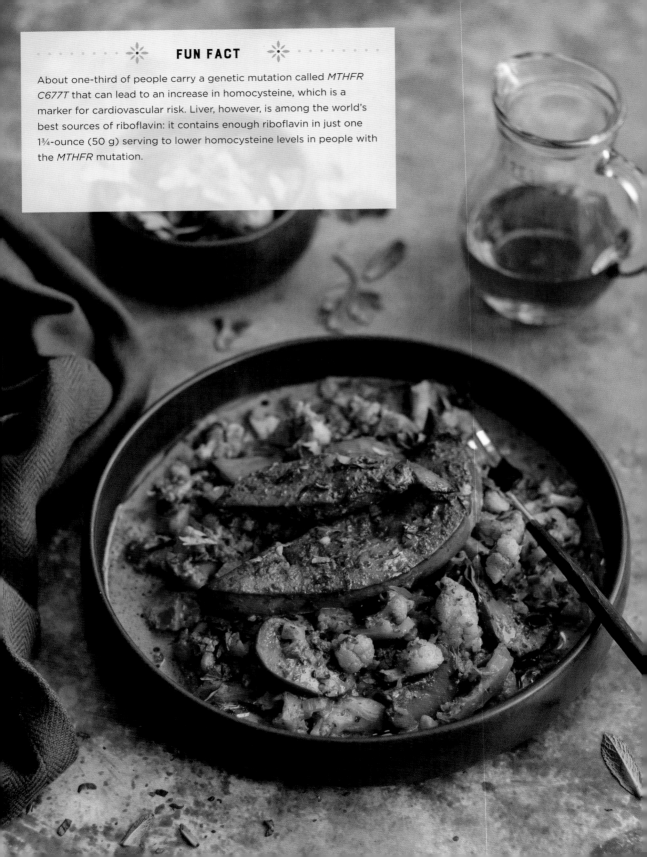

SERVINGS:
4

HANDS-ON TIME:
20 minutes

OVERALL TIME:
20 minutes
+ marinating
and soaking

HARISSA LAMB LIVERS

If you're looking for new ways to include more nutrient-dense organ meats into your diet, this dish is for you.

1.1 pounds (500 g) lamb livers, cut into about ½-inch (1 cm) slices

Enough filtered water to soak the livers

1 tablespoon (15 ml) red wine vinegar or fresh lemon juice

MARINADE

5 teaspoons (13 g/0.5 oz) Harissa Spice Mix (page 198)

Pinch of salt and black pepper

¼ cup (60 ml) extra-virgin avocado oil or ghee

SKILLET

½ small (30 g/1.1 oz) red onion, sliced

2 cups (140 g/5 oz) sliced brown mushrooms

1 small head (400 g/10.6 oz) cauliflower, cut into small florets

1 cup (240 ml) chicken stock or bone broth

1 cup (240 ml) goat's cream or heavy whipping cream

1 tablespoon (15 ml) fresh lemon juice

2 tablespoons (6 g/0.2 oz) chopped fresh mint

2 tablespoons (8 g/0.3 oz) chopped fresh parsley

① Place the livers in a bowl and add the water and vinegar. Cover and refrigerate to soak overnight. Drain the water from the livers and pat dry using a paper towel.

② To make the marinade: Place the harissa, salt, pepper, and olive oil in a bowl and add the livers. Place in the fridge and marinate for at least 30 minutes or up to 2 hours.

③ To make the skillet: Heat a large skillet over medium-high heat and add the marinated livers in a single layer. You will have some leftover oil marinade in the bowl; reserve this for cooking the aromatics. Cook the livers for 1 to 2 minutes per side (do not overcook) and then transfer to a plate and keep warm.

④ Use a kitchen towel to clean the skillet in which you cooked the livers (this will prevent any pieces from burning). Grease with the leftover marinade and add the onion. Cook for 5 to 7 minutes, then add the mushrooms and cook for 5 minutes. Add the cauliflower and chicken stock and cover with a lid. Cook over medium heat until the cauliflower is tender, 10 to 12 minutes. Add the cream and cook for 2 to 3 minutes.

⑤ Add the lemon juice and herbs and remove from the heat. Season to taste. Add back the livers and gently heat through for just a minute. Serve warm or refrigerate for up to 4 days.

NUTRITION FACTS PER SERVING:

Total carbs: 12.5 g	Fat: 44.6 g (of which saturated: 19.3 g)	SAT / MUFA / PUFA (%): 43, 47, 10
Fiber: 3 g	Calories: 578 kcal	Omega-6/3 ratio: 2.3
Net Carbs: 9.5 g	Macronutrient ratio: Calories from carbs (7%), protein (22%), fat (71%)	
Protein: 31.3 g		

SLOW-COOKED VENISON BOURGUIGNON

We've given the classic French dish a keto-friendly makeover! The traditional beef has been replaced with juicy venison, which is slow-cooked with fragrant aromatics, earthy mushrooms, and a dry, juicy red wine. Why no beef? Venison is one of the leanest forms of red meat, and using it allows you to "control your fats," so to speak, adding extra-virgin olive oil, ghee, or tallow as you so choose. This also means that what looks like an indulgent meal is actually one of our lightest.

BOUQUET GARNI

4 sprigs fresh parsley

4 sprigs fresh thyme

1 teaspoon peppercorns

4 whole cloves

3 bay leaves

STEW

¼ cup (60 ml) extra-virgin avocado oil or ghee, divided

2 pounds (900 g) venison, cut into 2-inch (5 cm) chunks

1 small (60 g/2.1 oz) red onion, sliced

3 cloves garlic, sliced

One 750 ml bottle dry red wine, such as burgundy

1 tablespoon (15 ml) unsweetened tomato purée

1 teaspoon ground turmeric

1 teaspoon salt, or to taste

½ teaspoon black pepper

12 ounces (340 g) sliced white mushrooms

¼ cup (60 ml) extra-virgin olive oil

TO SERVE

Green Cauli-Mash (page 157) or Cauli-Rice (page 166)

① To make the bouquet garni: Place all the herbs and aromatics in a piece of cheesecloth and tie with a piece of unwaxed kitchen string.

② To make the stew: Heat a Dutch oven or a heavy-bottomed pot greased with 2 tablespoons (30 ml) of the avocado oil. Fry the venison chunks in batches over medium-high heat until golden brown, about 5 minutes. Remove the chunks from the pot and place in a bowl.

③ Lower the heat, add the onion, and cook for 5 minutes. Add the garlic and cook for 1 minute. Return the venison to the pot. Add the red wine, tomato purée, turmeric, salt, and pepper. Bring to a boil and mix well with a spatula, scraping the caramelized cooking juices from the bottom of the pot. Add the bouquet garni and mushrooms, cover with a lid, and cook for 3 to 3½ hours over low heat. When the meat is tender, remove from the heat.

④ Use a slotted spoon to remove the bouquet garni, then transfer all of the meat to a bowl while leaving some mushrooms and aromatics in the pot. Add the olive oil, then use an immersion blender to process until smooth and creamy. Cook for a few minutes to reduce the sauce and thicken. Add back the meat mixture and gently stir to combine.

⑤ Serve with cauli-mash or cauli-rice.

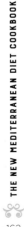

THE NEW MEDITERRANEAN DIET COOKBOOK

NUTRITION FACTS PER SERVING:

Total carbs: 7.2 g	Fat: 22.6 g (of which saturated: 3.3 g)	SAT / MUFA / PUFA (%): 15, 72, 13
Fiber: 1.1 g	Calories: 462 kcal	Omega-6: 2.4 g
Net Carbs: 6.1 g	Macronutrient ratio: Calories from carbs (7%), protein (38%), fat (55%)	
Protein: 34.5 g		

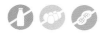

CRISPY SPICED DUCK & VEG TRAY BAKE

Duck legs get perfectly crisp in the oven, surrounded by winter vegetables roasted in the rendered duck fat. Go ahead. Indulge and live long! Duck is rich in thyroid-supporting selenium and has nice thick skin that's an excellent source of glycine, with a glycine to methionine ratio of 8:1. This is interesting because a higher glycine to methionine ratio diet has been shown in rodents to increase longevity.

SPICED DUCK

2 duck legs or 4 duck drumsticks (450 g/1 lb)

Pinch of salt and black pepper

1 clove garlic, minced

¼ teaspoon ground ginger

¼ teaspoon ground cumin

¼ teaspoon ground coriander

¼ teaspoon paprika

¼ teaspoon ground turmeric

¼ teaspoon black pepper

⅛ teaspoon cayenne pepper

⅛ teaspoon ground cardamom

3 tablespoons (45 ml) extra-virgin avocado oil or ghee

VEGETABLES

3 cups (250 g/8.8 oz) halved and trimmed Brussels sprouts

5.3 ounces (150 g) chopped cavolo nero kale, hard stems removed

Pinch of salt and black pepper

① Preheat the oven to 355°F (180°C) fan assisted or 400°F (200°C) conventional.

② To make the duck: Score the duck legs with a sharp knife and place in a bowl. Rub all over with the salt, pepper, and garlic. Combine the remaining spices in a small bowl and sprinkle all over the duck legs. Place the duck, skin-side up, on a baking tray and drizzle with avocado oil. Cook for about 1 hour and 10 minutes.

③ To make the vegetables: Remove the tray from the oven and use tongs to transfer the duck legs to a plate. Add the vegetables to the tray and toss in the rendered duck fat. Sprinkle with salt and pepper. Add back the duck legs and return the tray to the oven. Cook for 15 to 20 minutes, until the vegetables are crisp-tender, tossing halfway to ensure even cooking.

④ Serve warm or let cool and store, covered, in the fridge for up to 4 days.

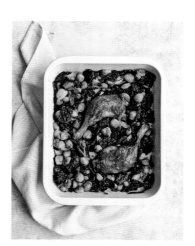

NUTRITION FACTS PER SERVING (1 DUCK LEG AND HALF OF THE COOKED VEGETABLES):

Total carbs: 16.2 g	Fat: 56.5 g (of which saturated: 14.8 g)	SAT / MUFA / PUFA (%): 26, 59, 15
Fiber: 7.6 g	Calories: 658 kcal	Omega-6: 6.8 g
Net Carbs: 8.6 g	Macronutrient ratio: Calories from carbs	
Protein: 27.3 g	(5%), protein (17%), fat (78%)	

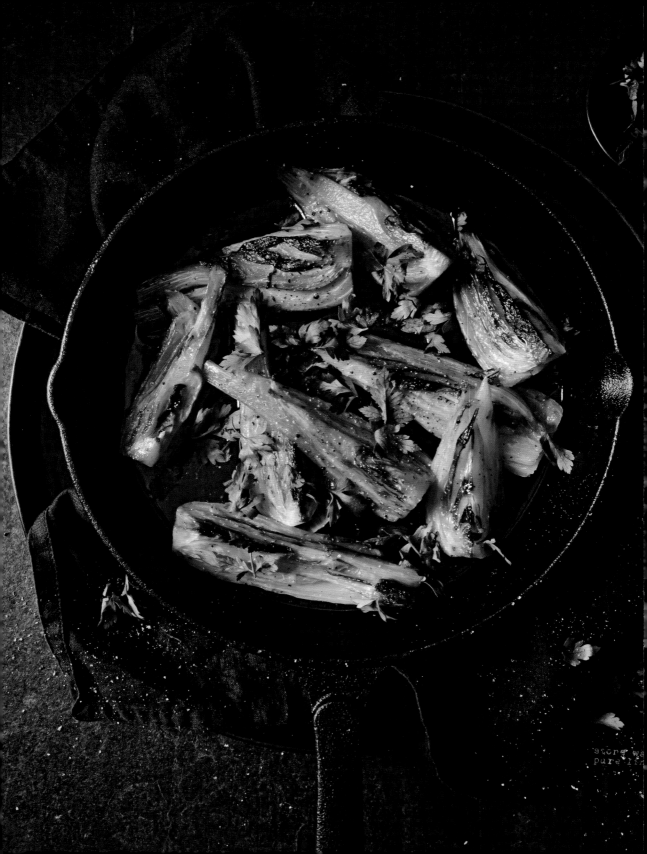

CHAPTER 7

SIDES

CAULI-RICE, THREE WAYS

Cauliflower rice is a keto staple, and for good reason: It's the most versatile of side dishes. Treat it like couscous or quinoa, or cook it in healthy fats and toss it with your favorite spices.

1 medium (720 g/1.6 lb) cauliflower

2 tablespoons (30 ml) extra-virgin avocado oil or ghee

Salt and black pepper, to taste

2 tablespoons (30 ml) extra-virgin olive oil, for topping

SPANISH RICE

½ small (30 g/1.1 oz) red onion, diced

½ medium (60 g/2.1 oz) red bell pepper, diced

1 small (85 g/3 oz) tomato, chopped

1 teaspoon paprika

½ cup (50 g/1.8 oz) sliced black olives

MOROCCAN RICE

½ small (30 g/1.1 oz) red onion, diced

½ teaspoon ground cumin

½ teaspoon ground turmeric

¼ teaspoon cinnamon

¼ teaspoon cayenne pepper

2 tablespoons (8 g/0.3 oz) chopped fresh parsley

2 tablespoons (14 g/0.5 oz) flaked or slivered almonds, for topping

ITALIAN RICE

1 teaspoon fresh lemon zest

1 tablespoon (15 ml) fresh lemon juice

2 tablespoons (17 g/0.6 oz) capers

½ cup (50 g/1.8 oz) green pitted olives, sliced

¼ cup (15 g/0.5 oz) chopped fresh herbs, such as parsley, basil, and thyme

① Run the cauliflower florets through a hand grater or food processor with a grating blade. Pulse until the florets resemble grains of rice.

② To make Spanish cauli-rice: Grease a large saucepan with the avocado oil. Add the onion and bell pepper. Cook over medium heat for about 3 minutes. Add the cauliflower rice and cook for 5 to 7 minutes, stirring occasionally. Stir in the tomatoes and paprika. Cook for 2 minutes, remove from the heat, and toss through the olives. Season to taste, drizzle with the olive oil, and serve.

③ To make Moroccan cauli-rice: Grease a large saucepan with the avocado oil. Add the onion and cook over medium heat for about 3 minutes. Add the spices and stir through. Add the cauliflower rice and cook for 5 to 7 minutes, stirring occasionally. Remove from the heat, stir in the parsley, and top with the almonds. Drizzle with the olive oil and serve.

④ To make Italian cauli-rice: Grease a large saucepan with the avocado oil. Add the lemon zest, lemon juice, and cauliflower rice. Cook for 5 to 7 minutes, stirring occasionally, until tender. Remove from the heat, and toss through the capers, olives, and herbs. Drizzle with the olive oil and serve.

⑤ Let cool and store in a sealed container in the fridge for up to 5 days.

NUTRITION FACTS PER SERVING (ABOUT 1 CUP [170 G] SPANISH/MOROCCAN/ITALIAN RICE):

Total carbs: 12/10.9/10.1 g	Fat: 16.2/16.2/16.2 g (of which saturated: 2.2/2.1/2.2 g)	Saturated / MUFA / PUFA (%): 14, 74, 12 / 13, 73, 14 / 14, 74, 12
Fiber: 4.9/4.3/4.3 g		Omega-6: 1.75 / 2 / 1.75 g
Net Carbs: 7.1/6.5/5.8 g	Calories: 198/194/188 kcal	
Protein: 4.1/4.5/3.8 g	Macronutrient ratio: Calories from carbs (15/14/13%), protein (9/9/8%), fat (76/77/79%)	

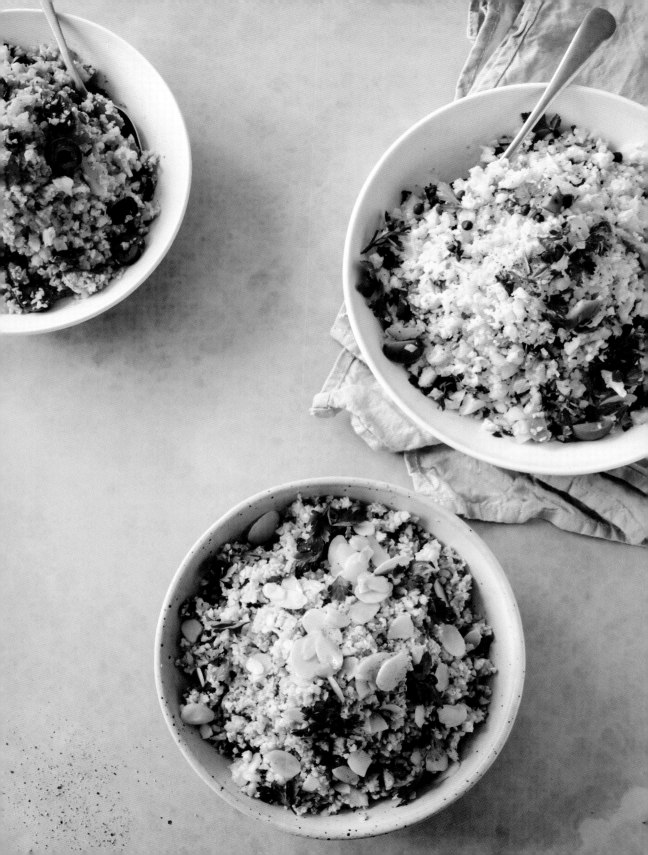

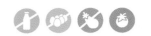

GREEN VEG & MACADAMIA SMASH

This emerald-green veggie mash is loaded with vitamins A, C, and K_1, other micronutrients, and it's extremely low in inflammatory omega-6 fats thanks to its macadamia base. Serve it as a side with fish and meat, alongside poached eggs at breakfast, or as a dip surrounded by colorful vegetable sticks for dunking.

⅔ cup (100 g) macadamia nuts

Enough water to cover and soak the macadamias

7 ounces (200 g) cavolo nero or kale, stalks removed and chopped

1 medium head (500 g/1.1 lb) broccoli, cut into florets, or broccolini

2 cloves garlic, crushed

¼ cup (60 ml) extra-virgin olive oil

2 tablespoons (30 ml) fresh lemon juice

4 medium (60 g/2.1 oz) spring onions, sliced

¼ cup (15 g/0.5 oz) chopped fresh herbs, such as parsley, dill, basil, or mint

Salt and black pepper, to taste

① Place the macadamias in a small bowl and add enough water to cover them. Soak for about 2 hours, then drain. Discard the water.

② Fill a large pot with about 1½ cups (360 ml) of water, then insert a steamer colander. Bring to a boil over high heat, then reduce to medium-high. Add the cavolo nero and cook for 6 minutes. Add the broccoli and cook for 8 minutes or until fork-tender. Remove the lid, let the steam escape, and let cool slightly.

③ Place the cooked vegetables in a blender or a food processor. Add the soaked macadamias, garlic, olive oil, lemon juice, spring onions, and fresh herbs (you can reserve some for topping).

④ Process to the desired consistency (smooth or chunky). Season with salt and pepper to taste and serve. To store, let cool completely and store in a sealed container in the fridge for up to 5 days.

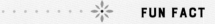 **FUN FACT**

Eating 15 to 30 macadamia nuts per day for 4 weeks can increase HDL and lower oxidative stress and inflammation.

NUTRITION FACTS PER SERVING (ABOUT ⅔ CUP/170 G/6 OZ):

Total carbs: 11.5 g	Fat: 22.6 g (of which saturated: 3.4 g)	Saturated / MUFA / PUFA (%): 15, 79, 6
Fiber: 5 g	Calories: 249 kcal	Omega-6: 1.1 g
Net Carbs: 6.5 g	Macronutrient ratio: Calories from carbs (10%), protein (8%), fat (82%)	
Protein: 5.3 g		

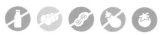

BRAISED FENNEL

Braised or roasted fennel is delicious with just about any kind of roast meat or fish. Slow cooking takes the edge off its crunchiness, brings out its inherent sweetness, and softens its licorice or aniseed flavor, transforming it into the most delicious, summery side dish.

2 large (500 g/1.1 lb) fennel bulbs

¼ cup (60 ml) extra-virgin avocado oil or ghee, divided

1 small (30 g/1.1 oz) shallot or red onion

1 clove garlic, sliced

4 to 6 thyme sprigs

1 small bunch (15 g/0.5 oz) fresh parsley, leaves and stalks separated

1 cup (240 ml) water

3 tbsp (45 ml) fresh lemon juice

Salt and black pepper, to taste

¼ cup (60 ml) extra-virgin olive oil, to drizzle

① Cut off the fennel stalks where they attach to the bulb. Reserve the stalks. Cut the fennel bulb in half, trim the hard bottom part, and cut into wedges.

② Heat a saucepan greased with 2 tablespoons (30 ml) of the avocado oil over medium-high heat. Sauté the shallot, garlic, thyme sprigs, parsley stalks, and hard fennel stalks for about 5 minutes. Add the water, bring to a boil, and simmer over medium heat for 10 minutes. Remove from the heat, set aside for 10 minutes, and then strain the stock, discarding the aromatics.

③ Preheat the oven to 355°F (180°C) fan assisted or 400°F (200°C) conventional.

④ Heat an ovenproof skillet greased with the remaining 2 tablespoons (30 ml) of avocado oil over medium-high heat and add the fennel wedges. Sear until caramelized, about 5 minutes, turning once. Pour the stock and the lemon juice over the fennel wedges, and season with salt and pepper. Loosely cover with a piece of aluminum foil. Bake for about 30 minutes. When done, the fennel should be easy to pierce with the tip of a knife.

⑤ Remove from the oven and scatter with the chopped parsley leaves and drizzle with the olive oil. To store, let cool and refrigerate for up to 5 days.

· · · · · · · · 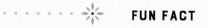 **FUN FACT** · · · · · · · ·

Fennel is great for your gut! Its natural compounds (including liquorice-tasting anethol) relax the gastrointestinal tract to promote normal bowel function. At the same time, fennel promotes the growth of good gut bacteria and kills bad gut bacteria, such as *Salmonella, E. coli,* and *Candida.*

NUTRITION FACTS PER SERVING:

Total carbs: 10.8 g	Fat: 27.4 g (of which saturated: 3.6 g)	Saturated / MUFA / PUFA (%): 13, 74, 13
Fiber: 4.2 g	Calories: 285 kcal	Omega-6: 3 g
Net Carbs: 6.6 g	Macronutrient ratio: Calories from carbs (9%), protein (3%), fat (88%)	
Protein: 1.8 g		

SIDES

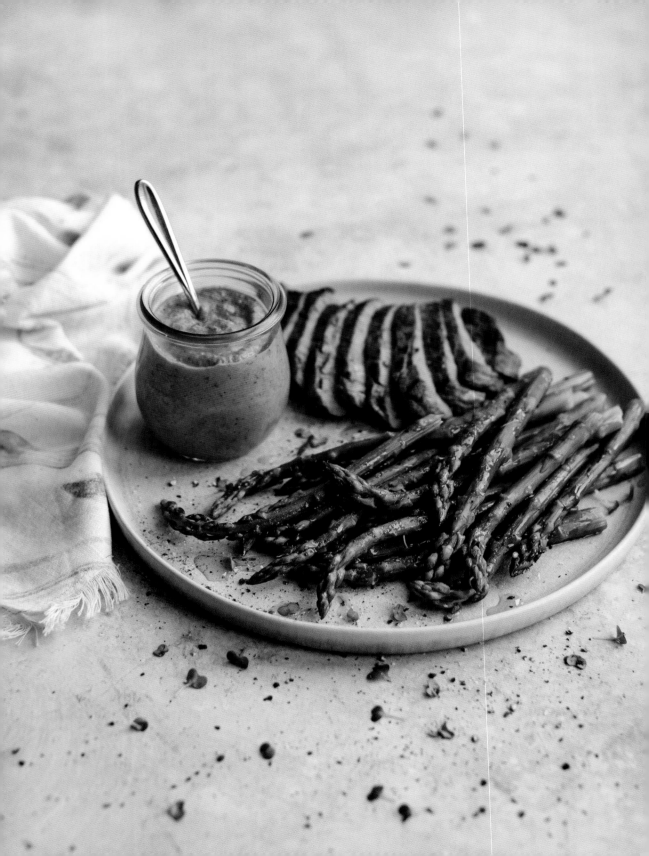

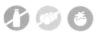 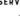

SERVINGS:	HANDS-ON TIME:	OVERALL TIME:
4	10 minutes	45 minutes

ROASTED ASPARAGUS WITH ROMESCO SAUCE

Romesco is a bold, creamy sauce that hails from Spain and uses roasted red pepper and tomato as its base. Add some MUFA-rich extra-virgin olive oil and hazelnuts, and you've got the perfect partner for roasted veggies, especially asparagus, which is gentle on the gut and loaded with prebiotic fibers to support the microbiome.

ROMESCO SAUCE

2 large (340 g/12 oz) red bell peppers or 7 ounces (200 g) cooked jarred red bell peppers

1 medium (100 g/3.5 oz) tomato, halved, or equivalent amount canned chopped tomatoes

½ cup (68 g/2.4 oz) peeled hazelnuts

2 cloves garlic, roughly chopped

2 tablespoons (30 ml) fresh lemon juice

About 2 tablespoons (8 g) chopped fresh parsley, basil, mint, or fennel fronds

¼ cup (60 ml) extra-virgin olive oil

Salt and black pepper, to taste

ROASTED ASPARAGUS

1.3 pounds (600 g) asparagus, tough ends removed

2 tablespoons (30 ml) extra-virgin avocado oil or ghee

Pinch of salt and black pepper

½ recipe Romesco Sauce (about 1 cup/240 ml)

① To make the sauce: If you're using fresh bell peppers, preheat the oven to 340°F (170°C) fan assisted or 375°F (190°C) conventional. Place the whole bell peppers and halved tomato on a baking tray lined with parchment paper and bake for 30 to 35 minutes. (If using canned chopped tomatoes, omit them here and add them to the food processor with the peeled peppers, below.) Remove from the oven and let cool for 10 minutes. Use a sharp knife to cut through the peppers and let the steam escape. Remove and discard the stems and seeds, then peel off the skins. (You can skip this step if you're using jarred peppers.)

② Transfer the peeled peppers to a food processor or blender. Add the remaining ingredients and process until smooth and creamy. You will only need half of the sauce per 4 servings. Leftover sauce can be stored in a sealed jar in the fridge for up to 1 week and served cold or warm.

③ To make the asparagus: Preheat the oven to 355°F (180°C) fan assisted or 400°F (200°C) conventional. Place the asparagus spears on a baking tray lined with parchment paper. Drizzle with the avocado oil and season with salt and pepper. Bake for 8 to 12 minutes (the exact time depends on the thickness of the spears).

④ Serve warm with the prepared Romesco sauce.

NUTRITION FACTS PER SERVING (ASPARAGUS · ¼ CUP/60 ML ROMESCO SAUCE):

Total carbs: 10.9 g	Fat: 19.2 g (of which saturated: 2.2 g)	Saturated / MUFA / PUFA (%): 11, 76, 13
Fiber: 5.1 g	Calories: 222 kcal	Omega-6: 2.2 g
Net Carbs: 5.8 g	Macronutrient ratio: Calories from carbs	
Protein: 5.2 g	(11%), protein (10%), fat (79%)	

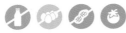

ROASTED CAULIFLOWER SHAWARMA

(CONTRIBUTOR: DR. UMA NAIDOO)

Even the word "shawarma" has a kick to it, don't you think? This recipe has almost as much spice as its contributor, Dr. Uma Naidoo, a triple threat in the food as medicine world. Dr. Naidoo is a professionally trained chef, a Harvard psychiatrist, and a nutrition specialist who founded the first U.S.-based clinical service for food as medicine! Serve her shawarma with roast salmon, chicken, or grilled halloumi, then take your meal to the next level by drizzling the whole thing with Tahini Dressing (page 200)!

1 large (1 kg/2.2 lb) cauliflower, cut into florets

⅓ cup (80 ml) extra-virgin avocado oil or ghee

1 clove garlic, minced

1½ teaspoons ground cumin

1½ teaspoons ground coriander

1 teaspoon ground turmeric

1½ teaspoons smoked or sweet paprika

½ teaspoon ground cardamom

1 teaspoon cinnamon

½ teaspoon cayenne pepper or to taste

1 tablespoon (15 ml) fresh lemon juice

1 teaspoon salt, or to taste

½ teaspoon black pepper, or to taste

2 tablespoons (30 ml) extra-virgin olive oil

Optional: chopped fresh herbs, such as parsley or cilantro, for garnish

① Place the cauliflower in a large bowl. In a small bowl, combine all of the remaining ingredients apart from the olive oil and optional herbs. Pour the spiced oil mix over the cauliflower and toss to cover on all sides. (Wear disposable gloves to prevent your hands from staining.) Marinate for 30 minutes or refrigerate to marinate overnight.

② Preheat the oven to 400°F (200°C) fan assisted or 425°F (220°C) conventional. Line one to two baking trays with parchment paper.

③ Add the cauliflower in a single layer on the baking trays. Pour any remaining marinade over the florets. Transfer to the oven and bake for 30 to 35 minutes, turning the baking dish halfway to ensure even cooking. Remove from the oven and drizzle with the olive oil. Garnish with fresh herbs, if using. Serve warm, or let it cool down, place in a container, and refrigerate for up to 5 days.

FUN FACT

Some people don't tolerate cauliflower and other cruciferous veggies because they contain a compound called raffinose that their digestive systems break down. However, you can buy a digestive enzyme called alpha-galactosidase that will digest the raffinose for you. That way you can enjoy your cauli and reap all of its health benefits, too.

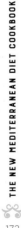

NUTRITION FACTS PER SERVING (ABOUT 1 CUP/ABOUT 150 G/3.5 OZ):

Total carbs: 10.3 g	Fat: 17.4 g (of which saturated: 2.3 g)	Saturated / MUFA / PUFA (%): 13, 74, 13
Fiber: 4.3 g	Calories: 198 kcal	Omega-6: 2.0 g
Net Carbs: 6 g	Macronutrient ratio: Calories from carbs (12%), protein (7%), fat (81%)	
Protein: 3.6 g		

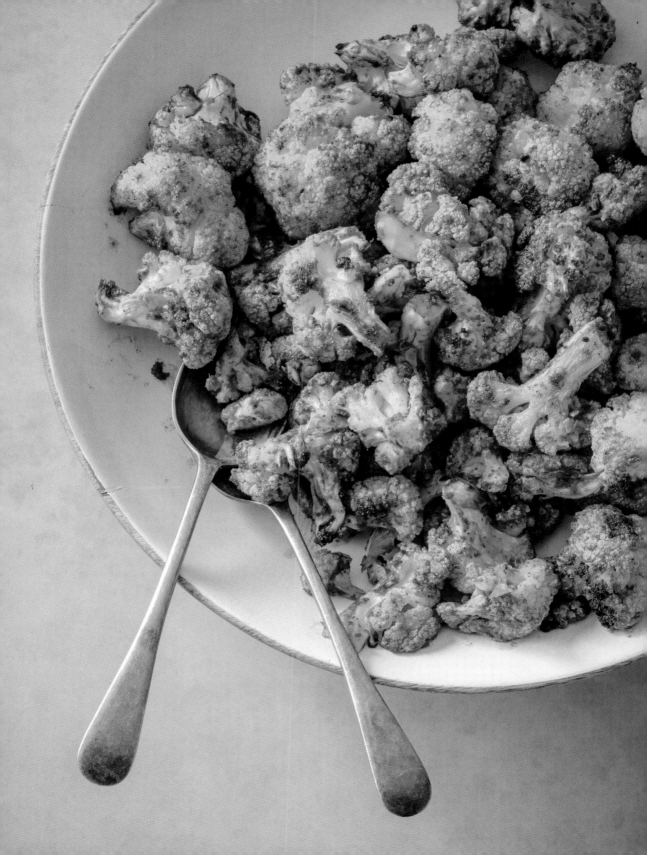

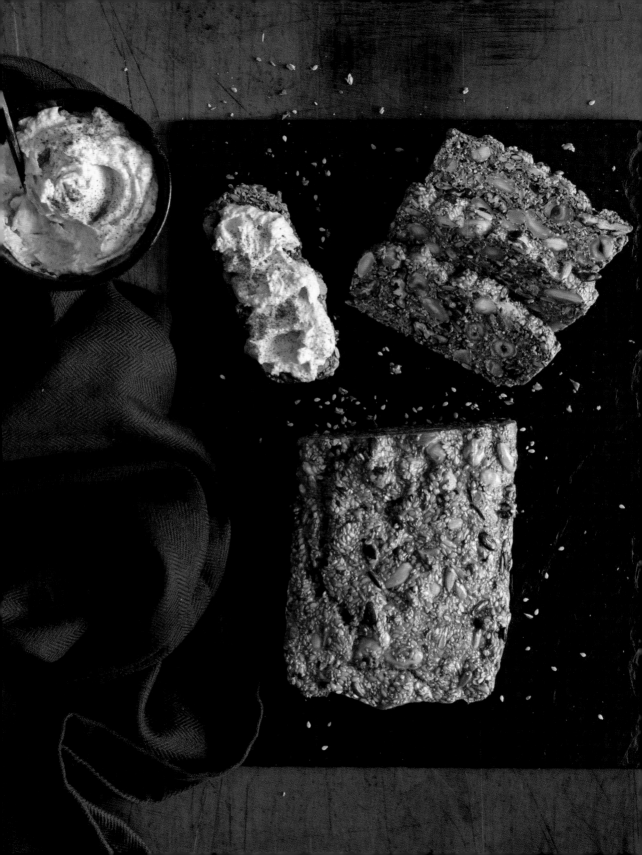

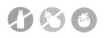

NORDIC STONE AGE BREAD

Our Nordic Stone Age Bread is made with a combination of nuts, seeds, eggs, and extra-virgin olive oil, and it's dense, satisfying, and nutritious. Any nuts or seeds will work here, so get creative and make it your own! Use it as a side for dips; to make packable sandwiches; or to serve alongside salads, soups, and stews. Try it with A+ Chicken Liver Pâté (page 76), Taramasalata (page 71), Goat's Cheese & Hazelnut Dip (page 77), or eat as a side with eggs.

½ cup (84 g/3 oz) flaxseeds

½ cup (76 g/2.7 oz) chia seeds

½ cup (72 g/2.5 oz) sesame seeds

¼ cup (32 g/1.1 oz) pumpkin seeds

¼ cup (35 g/1.2 oz) sunflower seeds

½ cup (72 g/2.5 oz) whole almonds, chopped

½ cup (68 g/2.4 oz) blanched hazelnuts, chopped

½ cup (50 g/1.8 oz) pecans or walnuts

1 teaspoon salt, or to taste

1 teaspoon coarse black pepper

4 large eggs

½ cup (120 ml) extra-virgin olive oil or melted ghee

① Preheat the oven to 285°F (140°C) fan assisted or 320°F (160°C) conventional. Line a loaf pan with parchment paper.

② In a mixing bowl, combine all of the dry ingredients. Add the eggs and olive oil and stir through until well combined. Pour the dough into the loaf pan. Transfer to the oven and bake for about 1 hour or until the top is crisp.

③ Remove from the oven and let cool slightly in the pan before transferring to a wire rack to cool completely before slicing. Store at room temperature for up to 3 days loosely covered with a kitchen towel, refrigerate for up to 10 days, or freeze for up to 3 months.

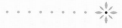

FUN FACT

Roasting nuts and seeds is a tricky business. In general, 285°F (140°C) is the threshold above which the antioxidants and omega-6 fats in the nuts become damaged. Macadamias are more resilient because of their low omega-6 and can be roasted at 300°F (150°C). Walnuts are the most sensitive and are best roasted at temperatures below 265°F (130°C). To demonstrate why we're so pro-macadamia, we offer you this statistic: If you roast equal amounts of macadamias and walnuts at 300°F (150°C) for 20 minutes, the macadamia will end up with one-thirtieth the oxidized omega-6 fats of walnuts! See what we mean?

NUTRITION FACTS PER SERVING (1 SLICE):

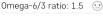

Total carbs: 8.5 g	Fat: 26.3 g (of which saturated: 3.2 g)	Saturated / MUFA / PUFA (%): 12, 58, 30
Fiber: 6 g	Calories: 290 kcal	Omega-6/3 ratio: 1.5 ☺
Net Carbs: 2.5 g	Macronutrient ratio: Calories from carbs (4%), protein (12%), fat (84%)	
Protein: 8.2 g		

SERVINGS:
6 tortillas

HANDS-ON TIME:
20 minutes

OVERALL TIME:
1 hour

SUPERFLAX TORTILLAS

These tortillas are so versatile, one might call them *super flexible* or even *hyper-plastic* (that's two puns, if you check out the fun fact). They're perfect for tortilla bowls, tacos shells, nachos, breadsticks, and even pizza crust!

1 packed cup (150 g/5.3 oz) flax meal

⅓ cup (40 g/1.4 oz) coconut flour

¼ cup (32 g/1.1 oz) ground chia seeds

2 tablespoons (8 g/0.3 oz) whole psyllium husks

1 teaspoon salt, or to taste

1 cup (240 ml) lukewarm water

2 tablespoons (30 ml) extra-virgin avocado oil or ghee

① Place all the dry ingredients in a bowl and mix to combine. (For ground chia seeds, simply place whole seeds into a coffee grinder or food processor and pulse until smooth.) Add the water and mix until well combined. Place the dough in the refrigerator to rest for about 30 minutes.

② When ready, remove the dough from the fridge and cut it into 4 equal pieces. You will make the remaining 2 tortillas using the excess dough. Place one piece of dough between two pieces of parchment paper and roll it out until very thin. Alternatively, use a silicone roller and a silicone mat. Remove the top piece of parchment paper. Press a large 8-inch (20 cm) lid into the dough (or use a piece of parchment paper cut into a circle of the same size). Press the lid into the dough or trace around it with your knife to cut out the tortilla.

③ Repeat for the remaining pieces of dough. Add the cut-off excess dough to the last piece and create the remaining 2 tortillas from it. If you have any dough left over, simply roll it out and cut it into tortilla-chip shapes.

④ Grease a large pan with the avocado oil and cook 1 tortilla at a time for 2 to 3 minutes on each side over medium heat until lightly browned. Don't overcook: the tortillas should be flexible, not too crispy.

⑤ Once cool, store the tortillas in a sealed container for up to 1 week and reheat them in a dry pan, if needed.

TIP: These tortillas are so versatile! Try these variations: ❄ Pesto Tortillas: 2 tablespoons (30 ml) any pesto (pages 198 to 199) ❄ Golden Tortillas: 1 teaspoon ground turmeric + 1 teaspoon ground cumin + ½ teaspoon ground coriander + ¼ teaspoon black pepper ❄ Garlic & Herb Tortillas: ½ teaspoon garlic powder + 1 teaspoon dried Italian herbs + 1 teaspoon onion powder

NUTRITION FACTS PER SERVING (1 TORTILLA):

Total carbs: 12.3 g	Fat: 17.9 g (of which saturated: 2.6 g)	Saturated / MUFA / PUFA (%): 15, 40, 45
Fiber: 10.8 g	Calories: 227 kcal	Omega-6/3 ratio: 0.4 ☺
Net Carbs: 1.5 g	Macronutrient ratio: Calories from carbs (3%), protein (14%), fat (83%)	
Protein: 6.8 g		

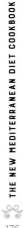

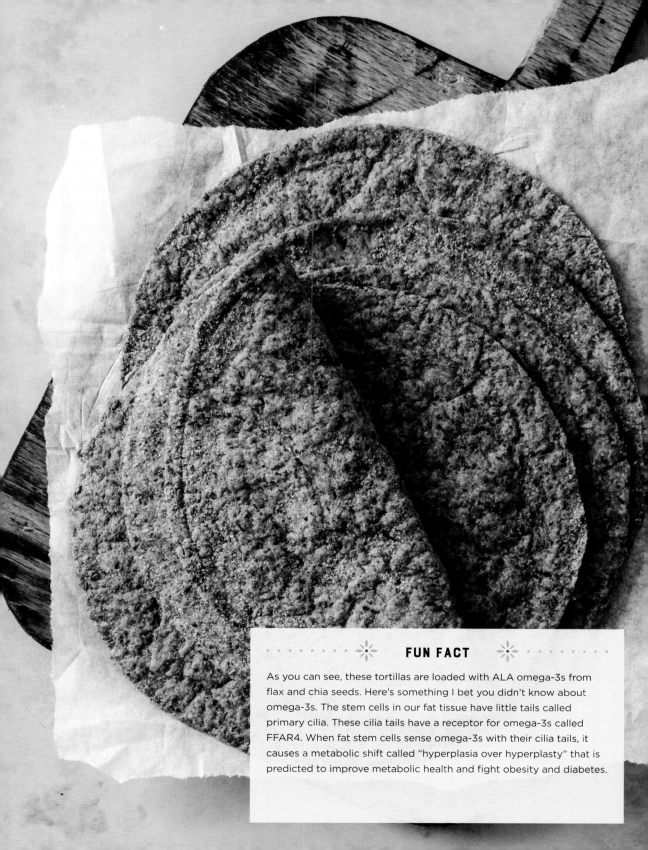

FUN FACT

As you can see, these tortillas are loaded with ALA omega-3s from flax and chia seeds. Here's something I bet you didn't know about omega-3s. The stem cells in our fat tissue have little tails called primary cilia. These cilia tails have a receptor for omega-3s called FFAR4. When fat stem cells sense omega-3s with their cilia tails, it causes a metabolic shift called "hyperplasia over hyperplasty" that is predicted to improve metabolic health and fight obesity and diabetes.

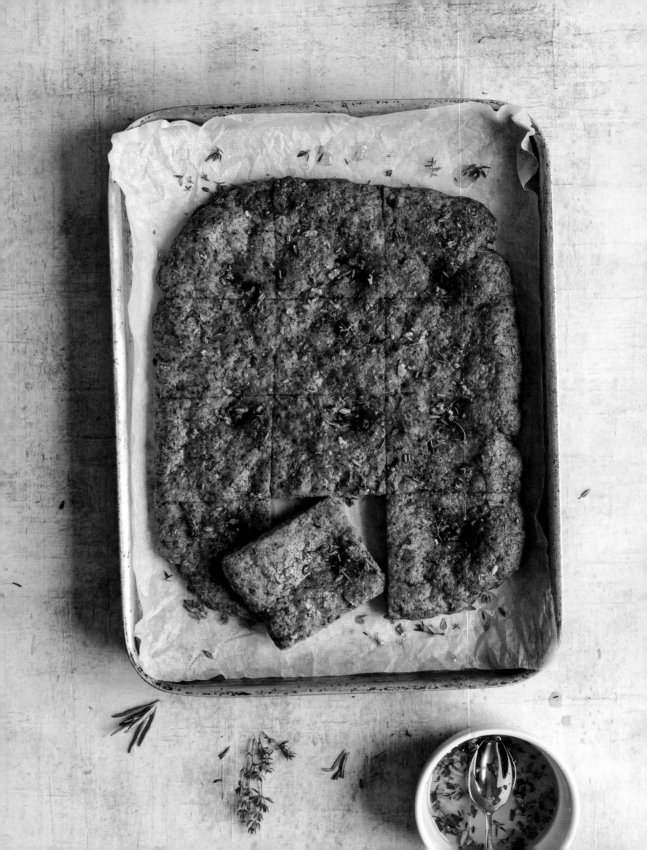

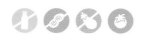

FOCACCIA

This soft, fluffy Italian-style olive oil bread is so richly infused with garlic and herbs that there's only room for 1 net carb! Beautifully crisp on the outside and soft inside, it is perfect for stuffing with your favorite sandwich fillings or to serve alongside salads and soups.

½ packed cup (75 g/2.7 oz) flax meal

½ cup (60 g/2.1 oz) coconut flour

¼ cup (32 g/1.1 oz) psyllium powder (ground psyllium husks)

¼ cup (32 g/1.1 oz) ground chia seeds

1 teaspoon salt

½ teaspoon ground black pepper

½ teaspoon baking soda

2 tablespoons (8 g/0.3 oz) chopped fresh herbs, such as rosemary, oregano, or thyme

2 cloves garlic, minced

½ cup (120 ml) extra-virgin olive oil

8 large egg whites

1 teaspoon apple cider vinegar

1 cup (240 ml) lukewarm water

① Preheat the oven to 285°F (140°C) fan assisted or 320°F (160°C) conventional. Line a baking tray with heavy-duty parchment paper.

② In a bowl, combine the flax meal, coconut flour, psyllium powder, ground chia seeds, salt, pepper, and baking soda. In another bowl, combine the herbs, garlic, and olive oil. In a third, large bowl, beat the egg whites until they create soft—but not stiff—peaks. Add the vinegar while beating (this will help them stay fluffy).

③ Add the lukewarm water and half of the herb-oil mixture to the bowl with the dry ingredients and process well with an electric mixer (reserve the remaining herb-oil mixture for topping).

④ Immediately after you pour in the water and herb-oil mixture, while mixing, add a quarter of the whipped egg whites to make the dough fluffy, mixing well. Then gently add in the remaining egg whites, mixing all the time.

⑤ Transfer the dough to the parchment paper–lined tray. Use your hands to flatten it into a rectangle, slightly more than ½ inch (1 cm) thick. Use your fingers to create small dimples in the dough, then pour over the remaining herb-oil mixture. Bake for 30 to 35 minutes. When done, place on a cooling rack for 5 minutes, then cut into 15 pieces (3 rows by 5 columns).

⑥ Store at room temperature covered with a kitchen towel for up to 3 days or freeze for up to 3 months.

NUTRITION FACTS PER SERVING (1 SLICE):

Total carbs: 5.6 g	Fat: 10.6 g (of which saturated: 1.8 g)	Saturated / MUFA / PUFA (%): 17, 58, 25
Fiber: 4.5 g	Calories: 128 kcal	Omega-6/3 ratio: 0.7 ☺
Net Carbs: 1.2 g	Macronutrient ratio: Calories from carbs	
Protein: 4.1 g	(4%), protein (14%), fat (82%)	

ROASTED EGGPLANT WITH TAHINI DRESSING

Spiked with homemade tahini dressing, this simple side only calls for a handful of ingredients, and it goes so well with Mediterranean mains such as grilled lamb and fish. If you needed another reason to try it: Eggplant gets its rich purple hue from the antioxidant nasunin, which also protects the heart, and nasunin levels actually increase when the vegetable is cooked.

3 medium eggplants (900 g/2 lb)

¼ cup (60 ml) extra-virgin avocado oil or ghee

Salt and black pepper, to taste

1 recipe Tahini Dressing of your choice (page 200)

1 tablespoon (9 g/0.3 oz) sesame seeds

Fresh parsley, to taste, for topping

Optional: chile flakes, to taste, for topping

① Preheat the oven to 410°F (210°C) fan assisted or 445°F (230°C) conventional.

② Cut the eggplants in half lengthwise and score the flesh in a crisscross pattern with a sharp knife. Brush with the oil, and then sprinkle with salt and pepper. Place on a baking tray, cut-side up, and roast in the oven for 30 to 40 minutes, until the flesh is cooked through and golden.

③ Place the eggplant halves cut-side up on a serving plate. Drizzle the dressing over, and sprinkle with the sesame seeds. Top with chopped parsley and chile flakes, if using. Try it with fish, steak, or on its own.

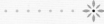

FUN FACT

MicroRNAs, little bits of transcribed genetic code, from plants can cross into the blood and alter human gene expression!

NUTRITION FACTS PER SERVING (½ ROASTED EGGPLANT • 2 TABLESPOONS [30 ML] CLASSIC TAHINI DRESSING):

Total carbs: 13.1 g	Fat: 23.5 g (of which saturated: 3.1 g)	Saturated / MUFA / PUFA (%): 13, 60, 27
Fiber: 6.2 g	Calories: 266 kcal	Omega-6: 5.7 g. Remember, tahini breaks the omega-6 rule because of its lignan antioxidants!
Net Carbs: 6.9 g	Macronutrient ratio: Calories from carbs (11%), protein (7%), fat (82%)	
Protein: 4.6 g		

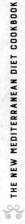

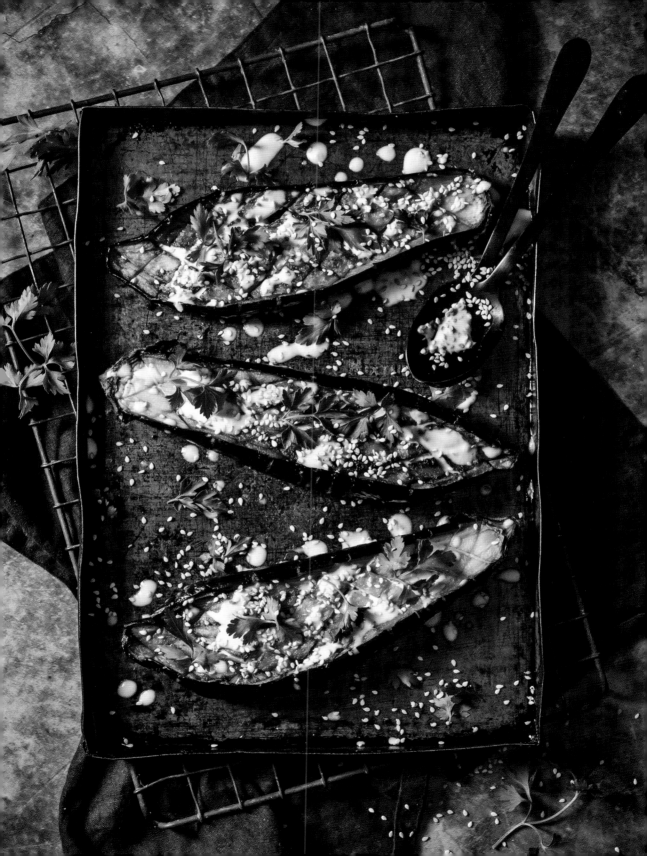

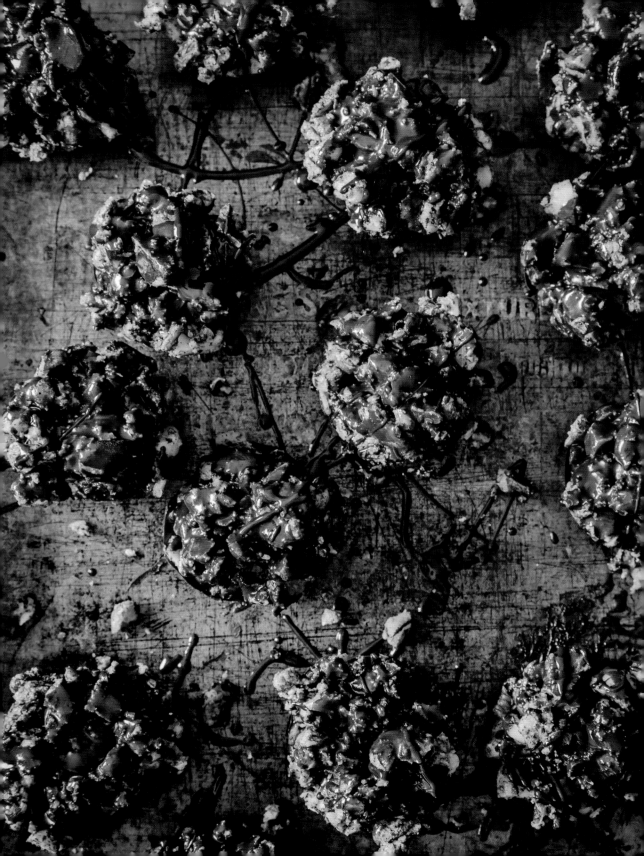

CHAPTER 8

DESSERTS

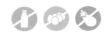

CHOCOLATE HAZELNUT "POWERHOUSE" TRUFFLES

(CONTRIBUTOR: DR. RUSSEL SWERDLOW)

This healthy take on a classic treat was contributed by Dr. Russell Swerdlow, an expert in Alzheimer's disease. He is credited with developing the "mitochondrial cascade hypothesis" of Alzheimer's disease, which is replacing older models in scientific textbooks. This newer model suggests that damage to mitochondria, the energy "powerhouse of the cell," leads to a domino chain of events and, eventually, dementia. Healthy brain aging is all about healthy mitochondria, which low-carb eating can help promote. Luckily, these bite-size treats are so full of Nutella flavor that there's just no room left for carbs!

FILLING

1¾ cups (236 g/8.3 oz) blanched hazelnuts, divided

½ cup (125 g/4.4 oz) coconut butter

4 tablespoons (57 g/2 oz) butter or ¼ cup (60 ml) virgin coconut oil

¼ cup (25 g/0.9 oz) collagen powder

¼ cup (22 g/0.8 oz) raw cacao powder

1 teaspoon vanilla powder or cinnamon

Optional: low-carb sweetener, to taste

CHOCOLATE COATING

2.5 ounces (75 g) 100% dark chocolate

1 ounce (28 g) cacao butter

Pinch of salt

① Preheat the oven to 285°F (140°C) fan assisted or 320°F (160°C) conventional.

② To make the filling: Spread the hazelnuts on a baking tray and roast for 40 to 50 minutes, until lightly golden. Remove from the oven and let cool for a few minutes.

③ Place 1 cup (136 g/4.8 oz) of the roasted hazelnuts in a food processor. Process for 1 to 2 minutes, until chunky. Add the coconut butter, butter, collagen powder, cacao powder, vanilla, and sweetener, if using. Process again until well combined. Place the dough in the fridge to set for 1 hour.

④ Reserve 12 hazelnuts for filling and crumble the remaining hazelnuts unto small pieces.

⑤ To make the chocolate coating: Line a baking tray with parchment. Melt the dark chocolate and cacao

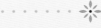

FUN FACT

Someone who has a mother with Alzheimer's is more likely to develop the disease, as compared to someone who has a father with Alzheimer's disease. This is because we inherit our mitochondria from our mothers.

NUTRITION FACTS PER SERVING (1 TRUFFLE):

Total carbs: 7.4 g	Fat: 27.9 g (of which saturated: 13.1 g)	SAT / MUFA / PUFA (%): 47, 48, 7
Fiber: 4.5 g	Calories: 283 kcal	Omega-6: 1.75 g
Net Carbs: 2.9 g	Macronutrient ratio: Calories from carbs (4%), protein (9%), fat (87%)	
Protein: 6.6 g		

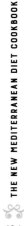

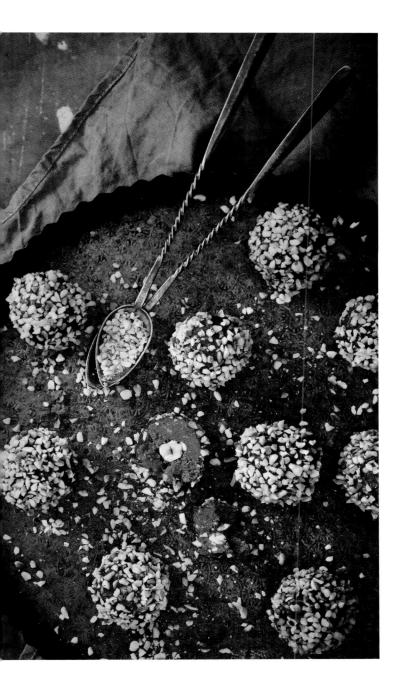

butter in a double boiler, or use a heatproof bowl placed over a small saucepan filled with 1 cup (240 ml) of water, placed over medium heat. Remove from the heat and let cool to room temperature before using for coating. Alternatively, use a microwave and melt in short 10- to 15-second bursts until melted, stirring in between.

⑥ Remove the dough from the fridge and use a spoon to scoop about 1 ounce (28 g) of the dough. Press one whole hazelnut into the center and use your hands to wrap the dough around to create a truffle. Place in the freezer for about 15 minutes.

⑦ Gently pierce each very cold truffle with a toothpick or a fork. Working one at a time, hold the truffle over the melted chocolate and spoon the chocolate over it to coat completely. Turn the toothpick as you work until the coating is solidified. Place the coated truffles on the lined tray and drizzle any remaining coating over them. Before they become completely solid, roll them in the chopped nuts. Refrigerate the coated truffles for at least 15 minutes to harden.

⑧ Keep refrigerated for up to 1 week or freeze for up to 3 months.

SERVINGS:	HANDS-ON TIME:	OVERALL TIME:
6	15 minutes	4 hours

BLUEBERRY PANNA COTTA

This deliciously creamy panna cotta, super low in omega-6, is delicately infused with vanilla and naturally sweetened with wild blueberries for an extra anti-inflammatory, antioxidant boost. Try to use wild blueberries—the cute little ones—in this summery dessert, if you can: They have at least twice as much antioxidant power as cultivated blueberries!

1 tablespoon (11 g/0.4 oz) gelatin powder

2 tablespoons (30 ml) water

2 cups (480 ml) goat's cream, coconut cream, or heavy whipping cream

2 cups (300 g/10.6 oz) wild blueberries, fresh or frozen, divided

½ teaspoon vanilla powder or 1½ teaspoons unsweetened vanilla extract

Optional: low-carb sweetener, to taste

① In a bowl, sprinkle the gelatin powder over the cold water. Set aside to let it bloom.

② Place the goat's cream, half of the blueberries (150 g/5.3 oz), and the vanilla in a blender and process until smooth and creamy. Alternatively, use an immersion blender.

③ Pour the blueberry cream into a saucepan. Gently heat; do not boil. Scrape the gelatin into the hot cream mixture together with the sweetener, if using. Mix well until all the gelatin has dissolved.

④ Divide among six 4-ounce (120 ml) jars or serving glasses and fill them about two-thirds full, leaving enough space for the remaining blueberries. Place in the fridge for 3 to 4 hours, or until set.

⑤ When the panna cotta has set, evenly distribute the remaining blueberries among the jars. Serve immediately or store in the fridge for up to 4 days.

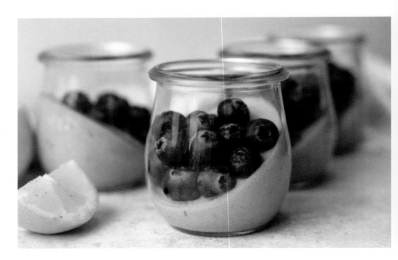

NUTRITION FACTS PER SERVING (1 JAR):

Total carbs: 8.3 g	Fat: 30.8 g (of which saturated: 19.4 g)	SAT / MUFA / PUFA (%): 63, 32, 5
Fiber: 1.3 g	Calories: 330 kcal	Omega-6: 0.8 g
Net Carbs: 7 g	Macronutrient ratio: Calories from carbs (9%), protein (5%), fat (86%)	
Protein: 3.7 g		

THE NEW MEDITERRANEAN DIET COOKBOOK

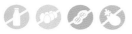

HALVA PROTEIN SLICES

Craving something sweet? Us, too. Here's our healthy take on a classic halva recipe—it's just as delicious, and it has none of the sugar used in the traditional version. Instead, it's packed with healthy fats and gut-healing collagen protein, so you can feel free to indulge!

¾ cup (180 g/6.4 oz) tahini

⅓ cup (85 g/3 oz) coconut butter

¼ cup (60 ml) virgin coconut oil

1 cup (100 g/3.5 oz) collagen powder

½ teaspoon vanilla powder or 1½ teaspoons unsweetened vanilla extract

½ teaspoon cinnamon

⅛ teaspoon salt

Optional: low-carb sweetener, to taste

① To soften the tahini and the coconut butter, place them in a small saucepan over low heat with the coconut oil. Remove from the heat and set aside to cool for a few minutes.

② Add the remaining ingredients and optional sweetener. Stir to combine, then pour the mixture into an 8 × 8–inch (20 × 20 cm) parchment-lined pan or a silicone pan, or any pan or container lined with parchment paper. Place in the fridge for at least 1 hour or until fully set.

③ Cut into 16 pieces and serve. To store, keep refrigerated for up to 2 weeks or freeze to up to 3 months.

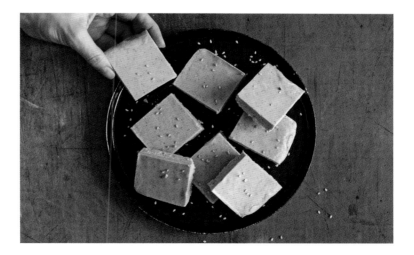

NUTRITION FACTS PER SERVING (1 SLICE):

Total carbs: 3.6 g	Fat: 12.3 g (of which saturated: 6.2 g)	SAT / MUFA / PUFA (%): 50, 26, 24
Fiber: 1.9 g	Calories: 149 kcal	Omega-6: 2.8 g. Remember, tahini breaks the omega-6 rule because of its lignan antioxidants!
Net Carbs: 1.7 g	Macronutrient ratio: Calories from carbs (5%), protein (21%), fat (74%)	
Protein: 7.6 g		

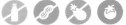

SERVINGS:
8 cream pops

HANDS-ON TIME:
10 minutes

OVERALL TIME:
3 to 4 hours

GOLDEN COCONUT CREAM POPS

This is a fun, refreshing, chilled-out version of a golden iced latte, a twist on the popular anti-inflammatory beverage. It boasts the anti-inflammatory power of turmeric, and it's also one of our lowest omega-6 recipes. You won't find any inflammatory fats here! Keep a batch in the freezer for a quick hot-weather treat.

1½ cups (360 ml) coconut cream

½ cup (120 ml) coconut milk

4 egg yolks

2 teaspoons (6 g) ground turmeric

1 teaspoon ground ginger

1 teaspoon cinnamon

1 teaspoon vanilla powder
or 1 tablespoon unsweetened
vanilla extract

¼ teaspoon ground black pepper

Optional: low-carb sweetener,
to taste

① Place all of the ingredients in a blender (including the optional sweetener) and process until well combined. Pour into eight ⅓-cup (80 ml) ice pop molds. Freeze until solid for 3 hours, or until set.

② To easily remove the ice pops from the molds, fill a pot as tall as the ice pops with warm (not hot) water and dip the ice pop molds in for 15 to 20 seconds. Remove the ice pops from the molds and then freeze again. Store in the freezer in a resealable bag for up to 3 months.

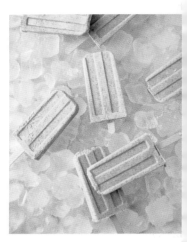

TIP: If a recipe calls for creamed coconut milk, make it a day ahead. To cream coconut milk, simply place the can in the fridge overnight. Open it the next day; do not shake before opening the can. Spoon out the solidified coconut milk and discard the liquids. One 13.5-ounce (400 ml) can will yield about 7 ounces (200 g) of coconut cream.

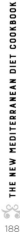

NUTRITION FACTS PER SERVING (1 CREAM POP):

Total carbs: 4.7 g	Fat: 20.9 g (of which saturated: 17.3 g)	SAT / MUFA / PUFA (%): 83, 15, 2
Fiber: 1.3 g	Calories: 209 kcal	Omega-6: <0.2 g
Net Carbs: 3.4 g	Macronutrient ratio: Calories from carbs (6%), protein (6%), fat (88%)	
Protein: 3.4 g		

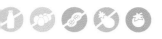

LEMON BERRY CREAM POPS

(CONTRIBUTOR: DR. DAVID DIAMOND)

These raspberry cream pops, coated in a thick layer of lemony goodness for extra zing, are an incredibly healthy snack. The recipe was contributed by neuroscientist Dr. David Diamond, who is also an outspoken advocate of low-carb eating for heart health. After battling his own high risk of heart disease with low-fat diets and exercise, his doctor told him he needed to start a statin drug. In his words, "Instead of going to the pharmacy, I went to the library." After reading a few thousand (!) scientific studies, he concluded that his heart disease risk could be remedied with a ketogenic diet. He now has a heart that could power a horse and is statin-free.

CREAM POPS

2 cups (480 ml) coconut cream

1 tablespoon (15 ml) unsweetened vanilla extract

Optional: low-carb sweetener, to taste

2 cups (300 g/10.6 oz) raspberries, fresh or frozen and defrosted

COATING

1⅓ cups (340 g/12 oz) coconut butter

¼ cup (60 ml) virgin coconut oil

Zest from 2 lemons, about 2 tablespoons (12 g/0.4 oz)

1 teaspoon unsweetened vanilla extract

① To make the cream pops: In a bowl, whisk the coconut cream with the vanilla and optional sweetener until smooth and creamy. In another bowl, crush the raspberries using a fork, then add them to the bowl with the coconut cream and mix to combine.

② Divide the mixture among eight ⅓-cup (80 ml) ice pop molds. Freeze until solid for 3 hours, or until set.

③ To easily remove the ice pops from the molds, fill a pot as tall as the ice pops with warm (not hot) water and dip the ice pop molds in for 15 to 20 seconds. Remove the ice pops from the molds and then freeze again.

④ Meanwhile, prepare the coating: Place the coconut butter and coconut oil in a small saucepan over low heat. Stir until smooth, remove from the heat, and add the lemon zest and vanilla. Let cool to room temperature.

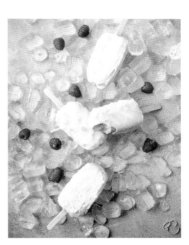

⑤ Remove the ice pops from the freezer, two at a time, and, holding the ice pops over the saucepan, use a spoon to drizzle the coating all over. Return to the freezer until fully set, about 10 minutes. Store in the freezer in a resealable bag for up to 3 months.

NUTRITION FACTS PER SERVING (1 CREAM POP):

Total carbs: 16.9 g	Fat: 51.1 g (of which saturated: 44.5 g)	SAT / MUFA / PUFA (%): 87, 11, 2
Fiber: 9.9 g	Calories: 520 kcal	Omega-6: 0.5 g
Net Carbs: 7 g	Macronutrient ratio: Calories from carbs (6%), protein (4%), fat (90%)	
Protein: 5.1 g		

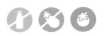

ALMOND PISTACHIO BISCOTTI

These twice-baked, crisp biscuits are delicious with coffee or tea. If you're craving something crunchy yet low-carb, these Italian-style cookies won't disappoint!

2 cups (200 g/7 oz) almond flour or hazelnut flour

½ packed cup (75 g/2.7 oz) flax meal

½ teaspoon baking soda

½ teaspoon ground nutmeg

½ teaspoon vanilla powder or 1½ teaspoons unsweetened vanilla extract

¼ teaspoon salt

1 tablespoon (6 g/0.2 oz) fresh lemon zest

2 large eggs

2 tablespoons (30 ml) extra-virgin olive oil

1 tablespoon (15 ml) unsweetened almond extract

1 teaspoon apple cider vinegar or fresh lemon juice

Optional: low-carb sweetener, to taste

⅔ cup (85 g/3 oz) unsalted pistachio nuts

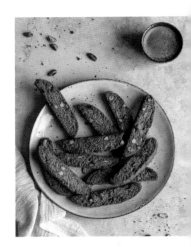

Mix well until a dough forms, then mix in the pistachio nuts.

③ Form the dough into a low, wide log shape, about 8 × 5 inches (20 × 13 cm). Place in the oven and bake for about 45 minutes. Remove from oven and let cool for 15 to 20 minutes. Using a sharp knife, cut into 12 slices.

④ Reduce the oven temperature to 250°F (120°C) fan assisted or 285°F (140°C) conventional. Lay the slices very carefully in a flat layer on the lined trays. Bake for 15 to 20 minutes, flip over, and bake for 15 to 20 minutes.

⑤ Remove from the oven and let the biscotti cool down completely to fully crisp up. Store in a sealed jar for up to 2 weeks.

① Preheat the oven to 285°F (140°C) fan assisted or 320°F (160°C) conventional. Line one or two baking trays with parchment paper.

② In a bowl, mix the almond flour, flax meal, baking soda, nutmeg, vanilla, salt, and lemon zest. Add the eggs, olive oil, almond extract, vinegar, and optional sweetener.

FUN FACT

Almond skins contain phytic acid, a plant anti-nutrient that can impair the absorption of minerals such as zinc, calcium, and iron. However, skinless almonds, also called "blanched" almonds, don't have nearly as much phytic acid. Almond flour is made from blanched almonds, which means that this recipe doesn't contain as much phytic acid.

NUTRITION FACTS PER SERVING (1 BISCOTTI):

Total carbs: 7.1 g	Fat: 17.7 g (of which saturated: 1.9 g)	SAT / MUFA / PUFA (%): 11, 51, 38
Fiber: 4.2 g	Calories: 207 kcal	Omega-6/3 ratio: 1.1 ☺
Net Carbs: 2.9 g	Macronutrient ratio: Calories from carbs (6%), protein (14%), fat (80%)	
Protein: 7.2 g		

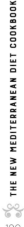

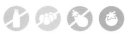

CREAMY NUT BUTTER CHOCOLATE CUPS

If you're missing store-bought chocolate peanut butter cups—and who can resist the heavenly combination of peanut butter and chocolate?!—we've got the solution. These low-fuss fat bombs are our healthy take on the treat, but with none of the sugar. The homemade nut butter adds a subtle sweetness that pairs well with ultra-dark chocolate.

5 ounces (142 g) 100% dark chocolate

⅓ cup (85 g/3 oz) Ultimate Nut Butter (page 79)

1 teaspoon cinnamon or vanilla powder

Optional: flaked salt, for topping

① Melt the dark chocolate in a double boiler, or use a heatproof bowl placed over a small saucepan filled with 1 cup (240 ml) of water, placed over medium heat. Remove from the heat and let cool to room temperature before using for coating. Alternatively, use a microwave and melt in short 10- to 15-second bursts until melted, stirring in between. Let it cool down.

② In a bowl, mix the nut butter with the cinnamon. Place about a teaspoon of the melted cooled chocolate in the bottom of a mini silicone mold and coat the sides of the mold by swirling it around. Repeat for all 10 molds. Place in the fridge for 10 minutes. This will help you get thicker sides and less chocolate will collect at the bottom.

③ You should have about two-thirds of the chocolate coating left in the bowl. Repeat the coating process one more time with another teaspoon: this will create a thicker cup to hold the nut butter filling.

④ Once you have prepared the chocolate cups, add the nut butter (about 1½ teaspoons per cup) and top with the remaining chocolate. Optionally, sprinkle each with a little flaked salt. Return to the fridge for 10 to 15 minutes. Store in the fridge for up to 2 weeks or freeze for up to 3 months.

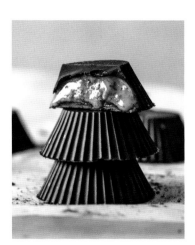

 FUN FACT

Cinnamon comes in two forms, Ceylon cinnamon and cassia cinnamon. Ceylon cinnamon contains two hundred times less coumarin, a compound that can poison the liver. For a person weighing 154 pounds (70 kg), all it takes is ½ teaspoon of ground cassia cinnamon to reach your tolerable daily intake of coumarin—but you'd have to consume a whopping 2 cups (250 g) of Ceylon cinnamon to reach that amount.

NUTRITION FACTS PER SERVING (1 CHOCOLATE CUP):

Total carbs: 3.7 g	Fat: 12.7 g (of which saturated: 5.8 g)	SAT / MUFA / PUFA (%): 46, 45, 9
Fiber: 1.9 g	Calories: 118 kcal	Omega-6: 0.7 g
Net Carbs: 1.8 g	Macronutrient ratio: Calories from carbs (5%), protein (8%), fat (87%)	
Protein: 2.8 g		

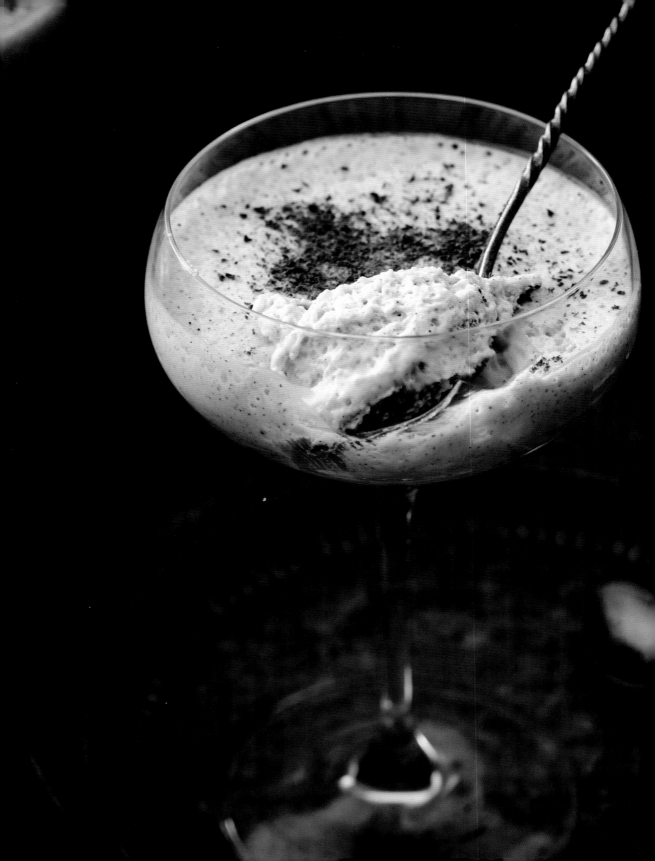

SPANISH CREAM

This unusual, airy, sugar-free dessert is much lighter than a mousse, yet still rich and complex in flavor. The best part? One serving contains less than 2 grams of net carbs! It's so gentle and soothing that it's perfect for winding down before bed. Plus, the gelatin is rich in glycine, an amino acid that may help improve sleep quality by acting on NMDA receptors in the brain.

3 large eggs

1¼ cups (300 ml) unsweetened almond milk, divided

1 tablespoon (11 g/0.4 oz) gelatin powder

1¼ cups (300 ml) goat's cream, heavy whipping cream, or coconut cream

1 teaspoon vanilla powder or 1 tablespoon (15 ml) unsweetened vanilla extract

1 teaspoon cinnamon, plus more for dusting

½ ounce (14 g) grated 100% chocolate, for topping

Optional: low-carb sweetener, to taste

① Separate the egg whites from the egg yolks. Place ½ cup (120 ml) of the almond milk in a small bowl, then add the gelatin and let it bloom.

② Place the yolks, cream, and the remaining ¾ cup (180 ml) almond milk in a heatproof bowl placed over a small saucepan filled with 1 cup (240 ml) of water, placed over medium heat, ensuring that the bottom of the bowl doesn't touch the water. Whisk while heating until the mixture is smooth and thickened.

③ Stir in the vanilla, cinnamon, sweetener (if using), and the bloomed gelatin. Cover with plastic wrap pressed to the surface, and chill for 30 minutes. At this point the mixture will look runny. Don't panic! This is absolutely normal. It will firm up.

④ In a bowl with a hand mixer, or in a stand mixer, whisk the egg whites until stiff, then fold them through the cooled custard. Divide among six serving glasses and chill until fully set, 3 to 4 hours. Sprinkle with the grated chocolate and, optionally, add the sweetener and a dusting of cinnamon. Store covered in the refrigerator for up to 5 days.

NUTRITION FACTS PER SERVING (1 GLASS):

Total carbs: 2.6 g	Fat: 23.2 g (of which saturated: 13.6 g)	SAT / MUFA / PUFA (%): 59, 36, 5
Fiber: 0.5 g	Calories: 245 kcal	Omega-6: 6 g
Net Carbs: 2.1 g	Macronutrient ratio: Calories from carbs (3%), protein (10%), fat (87%)	
Protein: 6.3 g		

DESSERTS

LEMON COCONUT CAKE

Birthdays and other special celebrations mean cake, and this one is sure to be the crowning glory of yours! You won't believe it when you taste it, but yes, this moist, zingy lemon cake is low-carb. Top it with fluffy whipped cream and finish it with crunchy toasted coconut flakes, then dig right in.

BASE

6 large eggs, separated

⅓ cup (80 ml) melted ghee or virgin coconut oil

1 tablespoon (15 ml) fresh lemon juice

Zest of 2 lemons (12 g/0.4 oz)

2 cups (200 g/7 oz) almond flour

½ cup (60 g/2.1 oz) coconut flour

¼ cup (25 g/0.9 oz) collagen powder

1 teaspoon baking soda

1 teaspoon vanilla powder or 1 tablespoon (15 ml) unsweetened vanilla extract

Optional: low-carb sweetener, to taste

TOPPING

½ cup (30 g/1.1 oz) unsweetened large coconut flakes

1 cup (240 ml) heavy whipping cream or coconut cream

¼ cup (60 g/2.1 oz) mascarpone, more heavy whipping cream, or coconut cream

½ teaspoon vanilla powder or 1½ teaspoons unsweetened vanilla extract

① Preheat the oven to 285°F (140°C) fan assisted or 320°F (160°C) conventional. Line a baking tray with parchment paper (or use a silicone tray). A square 8 × 8–inch (20 × 20 cm) or a rectangular tray of similar size will work best.

② To make the base: Whisk the egg whites in a bowl until stiff peaks form. In a separate bowl, whisk the egg yolks, melted ghee, lemon juice, and lemon zest. In a third bowl, mix the almond flour, coconut flour, collagen, baking soda, vanilla and optional sweetener.

③ Add the whisked egg yolk–ghee mixture into the dry mixture and combine well. Gently fold in the egg whites, trying not to deflate them.

④ Pour into the baking tray. Bake for 35 to 40 minutes, until lightly golden on top and set inside. Remove from the oven and let cool completely before adding the topping.

⑤ To make the topping: Preheat the oven to 350°F (175°C) fan assisted or 380°F (195°C) conventional. Place the coconut flakes on a baking tray and bake for 2 to 3 minutes. Remove from the oven and set aside to cool.

⑥ Once the cake is cool, place the cream, mascarpone, and vanilla in a bowl. Whip until soft peaks form. Spread on top of the cooled cake and top with the toasted coconut flakes.

⑦ To store, refrigerate for up to 5 days or freeze for up to 3 months. Coconut flakes will soften in the fridge. If you want to keep them crunchy, sprinkle on top of each slice before serving.

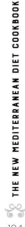

THE NEW MEDITERRANEAN DIET COOKBOOK

NUTRITION FACTS PER SERVING (1 SLICE):

Total carbs: 8.3 g	Fat: 38.6 g (of which saturated: 17.8 g)	SAT / MUFA / PUFA (%): 46, 39, 15
Fiber: 4.1 g	Calories: 432 kcal	Omega-6/3 ratio: 2.0 ☺
Net Carbs: 4.2 g	Macronutrient ratio: Calories from carbs (4%), protein (13%), fat (83%)	
Protein: 13.6 g		

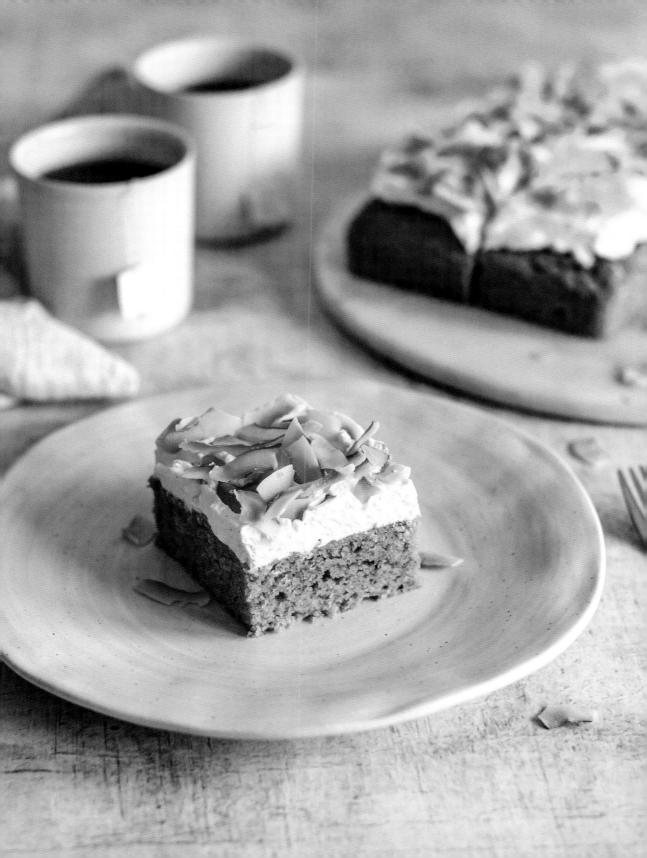

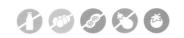

SERVINGS:
18 mini clusters

HANDS-ON TIME:
15 minutes

OVERALL TIME:
35 minutes

CHOLESTEROL CARING NUT CLUSTERS

Flavored with warming cinnamon, vanilla, and dark chocolate, these crunchy, sugar-free granola clusters are the perfect bite-size treat. And they can even help to improve cholesterol! The particular unsaturated fats in these nuts increase the number of LDL uptake receptors on the liver so LDL doesn't linger in the blood. Plus, the broad spectrum of polyphenol antioxidants scattered throughout all of these ingredients decrease oxidative stress and damage to LDL. That's a win!

CLUSTER BASE

1 cup (134 g/4.7 oz) macadamia nuts

1 cup (100 g/3.5 oz) pecan halves

½ cup (62 g/2.2 oz) pistachios

¼ cup (63 g/2.2 oz) tahini or coconut butter (although tahini is preferable)

1 large egg

1 teaspoon vanilla powder

2 teaspoons (5 g) cinnamon

TOPPING

2 ounces (57 g) dark chocolate

1 tablespoon (15 ml) virgin coconut oil or cacao butter

Pinch of flaked salt

① Preheat the oven to 285°F (140°C) fan assisted or 320°F (160°C) conventional.

② To make the cluster base: Roughly chop the nuts or place in a food processor and pulse until chopped but still chunky. Add the remaining base ingredients. Press the "dough" into 18 mini muffin cups and bake for 15 to 20 minutes, until crispy. Remove from the oven and allow to cool completely. Just before adding the chocolate topping, place them in the freezer for 5 to 10 minutes.

③ Meanwhile, make the topping: Melt the dark chocolate and coconut oil in a double boiler, or use a heatproof bowl placed over a small saucepan filled with 1 cup (240 ml) of water, placed over medium heat. Let cool to room temperature. Alternatively, use a microwave and melt in short 10- to 15-second bursts until melted, stirring in between.

④ Top the cooled clusters with the melted dark chocolate and flaked salt. Store in a sealed container in the fridge for up to 2 weeks or freeze for up to 3 months.

TIP: To make the clusters shelf-stable with no need for refrigeration, use cacao butter instead of coconut oil.

NUTRITION FACTS PER SERVING (1 MINI CLUSTER):

Total carbs: 4.2 g	Fat: 15.6 g (of which saturated: 3.4 g)	Saturated / MUFA / PUFA (%): 21, 61, 18
Fiber: 2.2 g	Calories: 157 kcal	Omega-6: 2.5 g. Remember, sesame/tahini breaks the omega-6 rule because of its lignan antioxidants!
Net Carbs: 2 g	Macronutrient ratio: Calories from carbs (5%), protein (8%), fat (87%)	
Protein: 3.2 g		

CHAPTER 9

BASICS

HARISSA SPICE MIX

2 tablespoons (14 g) ground cumin

4 teaspoons (10 g) paprika

4 teaspoons (9 g) ground turmeric

2 teaspoons (4 g) ground coriander

2 teaspoons (5 g) chili powder

1 teaspoon garlic powder

1 teaspoon ground caraway seeds

½ teaspoon cayenne powder

① Place all of the ingredients in a jar. Seal and shake well to combine. Store in a sealed jar at room temperature for up to 6 months.

SERVINGS: Makes about 7 tablespoons (46 g/1.5 oz)

BLENDER MARINARA SAUCE

1 cup (150 g/5.3 oz) chopped tomatoes

½ cup (20 g/0.7 oz) fresh basil leaves

2 cloves garlic

1 small (30 g/1.1 oz) red onion

¼ cup (60 g/2.1 oz) tomato paste

¼ cup (60 ml) extra-virgin olive oil

Salt and black pepper to taste

① Place the ingredients in a blender. Pulse until smooth. Store in the fridge in a sealed jar for up to 1 week.

SERVINGS: Makes about 1¼ cups (300 ml)

NUTRITION FACTS PER SERVING (¼ CUP/60 ML):

Total carbs: 2.9 g	
Fiber: 0.7 g	
Net Carbs: 2.2 g	
Protein: 0.6 g	
Fat: 10.9 g (of which saturated: 1.5 g)	
Energy: 110 kcal	
Calories from carbs (8%), protein (2%), fat (90%)	
SAT / MUFA / PUFA (%): 14, 76, 10	
Omega-6: 1.1 g	

PESTO, FIVE WAYS

MACADAMIA BASIL PESTO

2 cups (30 g/1.1 oz) fresh basil leaves

½ cup (67 g/2.4 oz) macadamia nuts

4 cloves garlic

1 teaspoon fresh lemon zest

1 tablespoon (15 ml) fresh lemon juice

½ cup (120 ml) extra-virgin olive oil

Optional: ⅓ cup (30 g/1.1 oz) grated Pecorino Romano cheese

Salt and black pepper

AVOCADO PISTACHIO PESTO

½ medium (75 g/2.7 oz) avocado

2 cups (30 g/1.1 oz) fresh basil leaves

⅓ cup (41 g/1.4 oz) raw pistachio nuts

1 tablespoon (15 ml) fresh lemon juice

4 cloves garlic

½ cup (120 ml) extra-virgin olive oil

Salt and black pepper

HAZELNUT ARUGULA PESTO

½ cup (56 g/2 oz) peeled raw hazelnuts

2 cups (20 g/0.7 oz) arugula

1 cup (15 g/0.5 oz) fresh basil or parsley leaves

4 cloves garlic

⅓ cup (80 ml) extra-virgin olive oil

3 tablespoons (45 ml) hazelnut oil

Salt and black pepper

BRAZIL NUT WATERCRESS PESTO

2 cups (30 g/1.1 oz) fresh basil leaves

2 cups (50 g/1.8 oz) watercress

⅓ cup (50 g/1.8 oz) Brazil nuts

¼ cup (32 g/1.1 oz) pumpkin seeds

2 cloves garlic

1 tablespoon (15 ml) fresh lemon juice

½ cup (120 ml) extra-virgin olive oil

Optional: ⅓ cup (30 g/1.1 oz) grated
Pecorino Romano cheese

Salt and black pepper

JALAPEÑO MINT PESTO

2 cups (30 g/1.1 oz) fresh mint leaves

½ cup (67 g/2.4 oz) macadamia nuts

1 jalapeño pepper (14 g/0.5 oz), seeds removed

2 cloves garlic

1 teaspoon fresh lemon zest

1 tablespoon (15 ml) fresh lemon juice

½ cup (120 ml) extra-virgin olive oil

Salt and black pepper

① Place all of the ingredients of your chosen pesto, except salt and pepper, into a blender and process until smooth. Season to taste with the salt and pepper.

SERVINGS: Makes about 1 cup (240 ml)

NUTRITION FACTS PER SERVING (1 TABLESPOON/15 ML MACADAMIA BASIL PESTO):

Total carbs: 1 g
Fiber: 0.5 g
Net Carbs: 0.5 g
Protein: 0.4 g
Fat: 9.9 g (of which saturated: 1.4 g)
Energy: 92 kcal
Calories from carbs (2%), protein (2%), fat (96%)
SAT / MUFA / PUFA (%): 14, 78, 8
Omega-6: 0.75 g

TIPS: Store your pesto in the fridge for up to 1 to 2 weeks. Each time you use the pesto, always remember to add a thin layer of olive oil on top before you place it back in the fridge. ❄ To preserve pesto for longer, spoon it into an ice-cube tray and freeze. Once frozen, store the pesto "ice cubes" in a resealable plastic bag in the freezer for up to 6 months.

BLENDER MAYONNAISE

2 large pasteurized egg yolks

2 teaspoons (10 ml) Dijon or yellow mustard

2 tablespoons (30 ml) apple cider vinegar

½ teaspoon fine salt

¼ teaspoon freshly ground black pepper

1½ cups (360 ml) avocado or macadamia oil

2 tablespoons (30 ml) lemon juice

Optional: 2 large capsules of probiotic powder

① First, make sure all the ingredients have reached room temperature. Place all of the ingredients except the oil, lemon juice, and probiotic powder in the small bowl of a food processor.

② Start the food processor and very slowly drizzle in the oil while the blade is running. Continue to pour the oil in slowly until the mayonnaise reaches the desired thickness. Some food processors have a small container with a hole specifically designed for this purpose so you can pour all of the oil into the container at once: the machine will drizzle it in slowly for you.

③ Once thick, add the lemon juice and blitz again for a few seconds to combine. Taste and readjust the seasoning if necessary. To make the mayonnaise last a few months, empty the probiotic capsules into the mayonnaise and mix well.

(continued)

④ Let the mayonnaise rest, uncovered, on the kitchen counter for 8 hours to activate the enzymes that will keep your mayonnaise fresh. You can then store it in the fridge in a sealed glass jar for up to 3 months.

SERVINGS: Makes about 2 cups (480 ml)

NUTRITION FACTS PER SERVING (1 TABLESPOON/15 ML MAYO):

Total carbs: 0.1 g
Fiber: 0 g
Net Carbs: 0.1 g
Protein: 0.2 g
Fat: 12 g (of which saturated: 1.2 g)
Energy: 108 kcal
Calories from carbs (0%), protein (1%), fat (99%)
With Avocado Oil
SAT / MUFA / PUFA (%): 10, 72, 18
Omega-6: 1.4 g
With Macadamia Oil
SAT / MUFA / PUFA (%): 18, 80, 2
Omega-6: 0.2 g

TIP: Add extra flavor to your mayo with one of these options: ❊ ¼–½ teaspoon ground turmeric + 1 teaspoon black pepper ❊ ¼–½ teaspoon smoked paprika + 1 tablespoon (15 ml) fresh lime juice ❊ ¼ teaspoon ground fennel seeds + ½ teaspoon fine fresh lemon zest ❊ 2–4 tablespoons (8–16 g) chopped herbs of choice

TIP: Drive down the omega-6 in your mayo by using macadamia oil (2% omega-6) instead of avocado oil (14% omega-6).

TAHINI DRESSING, THREE WAYS

CLASSIC TAHINI DRESSING

6 tablespoons (96 g/3.4 oz) tahini
1 tablespoon (15 ml) lemon juice
2 cloves garlic, minced
2 tablespoons (30 ml) extra-virgin olive oil
2 to 4 tablespoons (30 to 60 ml) filtered water
Pinch each of salt and pepper

GOLDEN TAHINI DRESSING

½ teaspoon ground turmeric
½ teaspoon ground cumin
½ teaspoon paprika
1 tablespoon (4 g/0.2 oz) chopped fresh cilantro

GREEN GODDESS TAHINI DRESSING

¼ cup (34 g/1.2 oz) macadamia nuts
½ cup (5 g/0.2 oz) loose basil leaves

① To make the classic tahini dressing: Add all of the ingredients to a small mixing bowl. Whisk using a balloon whisk until smooth and creamy. Store in a sealed jar in the fridge for up to 1 week.

② To make the golden tahini dressing: Follow the Classic Tahini Dressing recipe and mix in the remaining ingredients.

③ To make the green goddess tahini dressing: Follow the Classic Tahini Dressing recipe but instead use a food processor, add the remaining ingredients, and blend until smooth.

SERVINGS: 6 (2 tablespoons/30 ml per serving)

NUTRITION FACTS PER SERVING (2 TABLESPOONS/30 ML CLASSIC TAHINI DRESSING):

Total carbs: 3.9 g	
Fiber: 1.5 g	
Net Carbs: 2.4 g	
Protein: 2.8 g	
Fat: 13.1 g (of which saturated: 1.8 g)	
Energy: 137 kcal	
Calories from carbs (7%), protein (8%), fat (85%)	
SAT / MUFA / PUFA (%): 14, 53, 33	
Omega-6: 4.7 g	

SAUERKRAUT, TWO WAYS

1 large head (0.9 kg/2 lb) cabbage

1 tablespoon (17 g/0.6 oz) salt

2 teaspoons (4 g) ground black pepper

ANTI-INFLAMMATORY GOLDEN SAUERKRAUT

¼ cup (28 g/1 oz) grated fresh ginger

¼ cup (28 g/1 oz) grated fresh turmeric or 1 tablespoon (9 g/0.3 oz) ground turmeric

1 tablespoon (5 g/0.2 oz) ground cumin

2 teaspoons (5 g) cumin seeds

8 cloves garlic, minced

SPICY KICKIN' SAUERKRAUT

1 large (150 g/3.5 oz) red onion, sliced

4 red chile peppers (57 g/2 oz), sliced and deseeded

1 tablespoon (6 g/0.2 oz) red chile flakes

2 tablespoons (11 g/0.4 oz) dried oregano

① Cut the cabbage into quarters and remove the hard cores. Discard any dry outer leaves. Slice the cabbage with a knife or use a slicing blade on your food processor. Transfer it to a large bowl; sprinkle with the salt and ground black pepper.

② Add the ingredients for the anti-inflammatory or spicy kickin' sauerkraut to the cabbage and mix well. Let the mixture sit for about 2 hours. Press down on and squeeze the cabbage to release as much of the juices as you can. Place the "sweated" cabbage in a 1-quart (950 ml) Fido jar (or use two smaller jars), leaving about 2 inches (5 cm) between the top of the cabbage and the top of the jar, and close it. Don't worry about the jar exploding: The fermentation gases will escape through the rubber lid without letting oxygen in, so there will be no risk of failure. Oxygen is what causes mold, so do not open the jar during fermentation.

③ Store the jar away from direct sunlight and ferment at room temperature, 60° to 75°F (16° to 24°C), for 3 to 5 weeks. When done, refrigerate and store up to 6 months or preserve for longer, **without opening the jar.** Once open, refrigerate the jar for up to 2 weeks. If you open the jar to "test" it for taste but want to keep it for longer than 2 weeks, cover with a lid again and leave it for 2 to 3 days at room temperature before refrigerating.

SERVINGS: Makes about one 1-quart (950 ml) jar

NUTRITION FACTS PER SERVING (¼ CUP/36 G/1.3 OZ):

Total carbs: 1.5 g	
Fiber: 1 g	
Net Carbs: 1.5 g	
Protein: 0.3 g	
Fat: 0 g (of which saturated: 0 g)	
Energy: 7 kcal	
Calories from carbs (53%), protein (35%), fat (12%)	

TIP: Add healthy fats to sauerkraut by drizzling over 1 to 2 tablespoons (15 to 30 ml) of olive oil per serving.

FURTHER READING

There was too much we wanted to fit into this book to include it all in the printed version. Scan this code to see the bonus features and extra material online! This is the twenty-first century, after all!

ACKNOWLEDGMENTS

We would all like to thank the very talented Jo Harding, without whom we wouldn't have so many beautiful pictures of our recipes, as well as Eleanor Stanton, for creating all the illustrations. We would all like to thank the amazing team at Fair Winds Press, who put so much hard work into making this book a reality. It's been an absolute pleasure working with all of you! Special thanks to Jill Alexander, Renae Haines, Heather Godin, Barbara States, Megan Jones, Megan Buckley, Jenna Patton, Karen Levy, Tim Griffin, and Janie House.

ABOUT THE AUTHORS

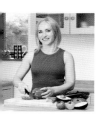

Martina Slajerova is a health and food blogger, mobile app creator, and best-selling author of ten cookbooks. She holds a degree in economics and worked in auditing but has always been passionate about nutrition, exercise, and photography. As a science geek, she bases her views on valid research and has firsthand experience of what it means to be on a low-carb diet.

After being diagnosed with Hashimoto's, an autoimmune disease that affects the thyroid, Martina had no energy and found it more and more difficult to maintain a healthy weight. The irony was that, like so many other people, she used to follow what is believed to be a healthy "balanced" diet based around whole grains and vegetables, and with limited amount of fats and animal products. That's when she decided to quit sugar, grains, and processed foods, and started following a whole foods–based ketogenic diet.

Since its launch in 2012, Martina's blog has helped millions of readers follow a healthy low-carb lifestyle and the KetoDiet app is now one of the best-selling health apps on the App Store and Google Play. Her book *The Keto All Day Cookbook* has been featured on ITV UK and her work has been featured in several international magazines, including *Women's Health*, *Glamour*, and *Cosmopolitan*.

Martina believes that a whole foods–based, Mediterranean-style keto diet that reflects our individual needs has the potential to help people break the endless dieting cycle while keeping their body nourished. No more hunger, no more cravings.

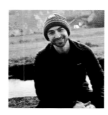

Dr. Nicholas Norwitz is a new shining star in nutrition science. This Ivy League Valedictorian obtained his Ph.D. at Oxford University in just two years and is now pursing his M.D. at Harvard Medical School. His research expertise is ketosis and brain aging; however, he has published scientific papers on topics ranging from neuroscience to heart disease to gastrointestinal health to genetics to bone health to diabetes.

Nick's passion for food as medicine is founded on personal history. At eighteen years old, he developed severe osteoporosis, a bone disease that crippled his promising running career. Next, Nick developed ulcerative colitis, an inflammatory bowel disease so severe as to cause him to lose 20 percent of his body weight in weeks and end up in the palliative care ward of a hospital with a heart rate in the twenties.

Through scientific self-study, Nick discovered his salvation in a ketogenic diet. He reversed his osteoporosis and colitis and is thriving! Nick is grateful for his apparent misfortunes. In his words, "The most remarkable part of my story is that it's not unique. The healthcare system isn't built to address metabolic diseases. For that, we need metabolic medicine rooted in nutrition. My lifelong goal is to help reform the system and educate people. Plus, I'd like to think being a patient has made me a more compassionate person."

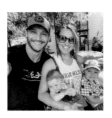

Thomas DeLauer is the founder of a successful corporate performance organization, specializing in combining optimized nutrition protocols and exercise and translating it into the best all-around performance in business and life. He is noted for his personal transformation from a 280-pound overweight corporate executive to being on the cover of health and fitness magazines worldwide. He is known internationally as one of the leading experts on the ketogenic diet and his YouTube channel garners over 5 million views per month and is one of the leading health education resources on the internet.

Thomas been highlighted in more than twenty magazines showcasing his transformation and has been featured on the cover of *Ironman Magazine*, *Muscle and Performance Magazine*, *Natural Muscle Magazine*, *ICON Magazine*, *Platform Magazine*, and *Ironman Japan*.

Residing in Central California, with his wife, son, daughter, three dogs, and old, trusty steed (horse), Thomas promotes a lifestyle of living as close to the earth as possible to obtain the best possible results while still achieving maximum performance in every possible area of life.

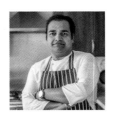

Rohan Kashid was raised in India and has been working as a professional chef in top restaurants and five-star hotels across Asia and Europe for over twenty years. As you can imagine, life as a professional chef isn't conducive to a healthful way of living. Rohan explains, "I'm surrounded by food sixteen hours a day. As head chef, I felt pressure to taste everything. I found myself obese and prediabetic."

But the scary thing, according to Rohan, is that "I didn't think much of it. It's becoming the norm. Back home, people just think of metabolic diseases, like diabetes and Alzheimer's disease, as parts of normal aging. I assumed that was in my future." That was, until a chance meeting with Nick in Oxford at Rohan's restaurant. The unlikely pair became good friends.

Cutting out carbs changed Rohan's life. He reversed his prediabetes, lost over 40 pounds, and discovered that "I've always been a perfectionist, and I now realize I can use nutrition to perfect myself." It's his missions to use his platform to shift public opinion. "People need to know that keto food can be, and should be, delicious without the craving!"

INDEX